MW01130211

TABLE OF CONTENTS

Top 20 Test Taking Tips

1. Carefully follow all the test registration procedures
2. Know the test directions, duration, topics, question types, how many questions
3. Setup a flexible study schedule at least 3-4 weeks before test day
4. Study during the time of day you are most alert, relaxed, and stress free
5. Maximize your learning style; visual learner use visual study aids, auditory learner use auditory study aids
6. Focus on your weakest knowledge base
7. Find a study partner to review with and help clarify questions
8. Practice, practice, practice
9. Get a good night's sleep; don't try to cram the night before the test
10. Eat a well balanced meal
11. Know the exact physical location of the testing site; drive the route to the site prior to test day
12. Bring a set of ear plugs; the testing center could be noisy
13. Wear comfortable, loose fitting, layered clothing to the testing center; prepare for it to be either cold or hot during the test
14. Bring at least 2 current forms of ID to the testing center
15. Arrive to the test early; be prepared to wait and be patient
16. Eliminate the obviously wrong answer choices, then guess the first remaining choice
17. Pace yourself; don't rush, but keep working and move on if you get stuck
18. Maintain a positive attitude even if the test is going poorly
19. Keep your first answer unless you are positive it is wrong
20. Check your work, don't make a careless mistake

Medical Terminology

Origin of medical terminology

Most medical terms derive from Greek or Latin, but there are a few English, French and German terms. If you break the Greek or Latin word into its root, prefix and suffix, then you can understand unfamiliar terminology. To avoid awkward pronunciation when there is no vowel between the root word and suffix, add an "o" to the combining form. For instance, add the suffix "metry" (meaning the measure of) to the root word for eye, "opt," to make the word "optometry". Examples of English terminology include: Epstein-Barr virus, HIV-positive, 100-ml sample, oxygen-dependent, or self-image. English words use a dash instead of a joining vowel. An example of French terminology is *grand mal* (the big sickness) for epileptic seizures. An example of German terminology is *mittelschmerz* (middle pain) for the discomfort of ovulation. French and German do not have convenient combining forms, so you must memorize them.

Prefix, root, and suffix

Medical terms have three parts:
- Root containing the basic meaning
- Prefix before the root that modifies the meaning
- Suffix after the root that modifies the meaning

Examples:
- Menorrhagia is excessive bleeding during menstruation and at irregular intervals. The prefix is meno, meaning menstruation. The root is metro, meaning uterus. The suffix is rrhagia, meaning a flow that bursts forth.
- Rhinoplasty is a "nose job". The root is rhino, meaning nose. The suffix is plasty, meaning reconstructive surgery.
- Antecubitum is the bend of your arm where the nurse draws blood. The root is cubitum, meaning elbow. The prefix is ante, meaning forward or before.
- Whenever you see an unfamiliar term, break it into its root, prefix, and suffix to understand its meaning.

Prefixes

Prefix	Meaning	Example
Ab	from, not here, off the norm	Abnormal
Ad	to, in the direction of	Adduct
Ante	prior to, in front of, previously	Antecedent
Anti	hostile to, against, contradictory	Antisocial
Be	make, aligned with, greatly	Benign
Bi	two, occurring twice	Bicycle
De	away, versus, reduce	Deduct
Dia	transverse, across	Diameter
Dis	contradictory, disparate, away	Disjointed

Prefixes - continued

Prefix	Meaning	Example
En	create, put in or on, surround	Engulf
Syn	by means of, together, same	Synthesis
Trans	across, far away, go through	Transvaginal
Ultra	extreme, beyond in space	Ultrasound
Un	opposing, antithetical, not	Uncooperative

The following is a list of common medical terminology *prefixes*:

A (without)
An (without)
Ante (before)
Bi (two)
Bin (two)
Brady (slow)
Dia (through)
Dys (difficult)
Endo (within)
Epi (over)
Eu (normal)
Ex (outward)
Exo (outward)
Hemi (half)
Hyper (excessive)
Hypo (deficient)
Inter (between)
Intra (within)
Meta (change)
Micro (minute, tiny)
Multi (numerous)

Neo (new)
Nulli (none)
Pan (total)
Para (beyond)
Per (through)
Peri (surrounding)
Poly (many)
Post (after)
Pre (before)
Pro (before)
Sub (below)
Supra (superior)
Sym (join)
Syn (join)
Tachy (rapid)
Tetra (four)
Trans (through)
Uni (one)

Suffixes

Suffix	Meaning	Example
-fication/-ation	manner or process	classification
-gram	written down or illustrated	cardiogram
-graph	a machine or instrument that records data	cardiograph
-graphy	the process of recording of data	cardiography
-ics	science or skill of	synthetics
-itis	red, inflamed, swollen	bursitis
-meter	means of measure	thermometer
-metry	action of measuring	telemetry
-ology/-ogy	the study of	biology
-phore	bearer or maker	semaphore
-phobia	intense, irrational fear	arachnophobia
-scope	instrument used for visualizing data	microscope
-scopy	visualize or examine	bronchoscopy

The following is a list of common medical terminology *suffixes:*

-ac (pertaining to)
-ad (toward)
-al (pertaining to)
-algia (pain)
-apheresis (removal)
-ar (pertaining to)
-ary (pertaining to)
-asthenia (weakness)
-atresia (occlusion, closure)
-capnia (carbon dioxide)
-cele (hernia)
-centesis (aspirate fluid off lung)
-clasia (break)
-clasis (break)
-coccus (berry-like bacteria)
-crit (separate)
-cyte (cell)
-desis (fusion)
-drome (run)
-eal (pertaining to)
-ectasis (expansion)
-ectomy (removal)
-emia (blood dysfunction)
-esis (condition)
-gen (agent that causes)
-genesis (cause)
-genic (pertaining to)
-gram (record)

-graph (recording device)
-graphy (process of recording)
-ia (disease condition)
-ial (pertaining to)
-iasis (condition)
-iatrist (physician)
-iatry (specialty)
-ic (pertaining to)
-ician (one that)
-ictal (attack)
-ior (pertaining to)
-ism (condition of)
-it is (inflammation)
-lysis (separating)
-malacia (softening)
-megaly (increasing in size)
-meter (measure)
-odynia (pain)
-oid (resembling)
-ologist (person that practices)
-ology (study)
-oma (tumor)
-opia (vision)
-opsy (view of)
-orrhagia (blood flowing profusely)
-orrhaphy (repairing)
-orrhea (flow)
-orrhexis (break)

Common medical terminology *suffixes* continued:

-osis (condition)
-ostomy (to make an opening)
-otomy (cut into)
-ous (pertaining to)
-oxia (oxygen)
-paresis (partial paralysis)
-pathy (disease)
-penia (decrease in number)
-pepsia (digestion)
-pexy (suspension)
-phagia (swallowing, eating)
-phobia (excessive fear of)
-phonia (sound, voice)
-physis (growth)
-plasia (development)
-plasm (a growth)
-plasty (repair by surgery)

-plegia (paralysis)
-pnea (breathing)
-poiesis (formation)
-ptosis (sagging)
-salpinx (fallopian tube)
-sarcoma (malignant tumor)
-schisis (crack)
-sclerosis (hardening)
-scope (visual device used for inspection)
-scopic (visual inspection)
-sis (condition of)
-spasm (abnormal muscle firing)
-stasis (standing)
-stenosis (narrowing)
-thorax (chest)
-tocia (labor, birth)
-tome (cutting device)
-tripsy (surgical crushing)
-trophy (develop)
-uria (urine)

Common word roots

The following is a list of common medical terminology *word roots:*

abdomin/o (abdomen)
acou/o (hearing)
acr/o (height/extremities)
aden/o (gland)
adenoid/o (adenoids)
adren/o (adrenal gland)
alveol/o (alveolus)
amni/o (amnion)
andro/o (male)
angi/o (vessel)
ankly/o (stiff)
anter/o (frontal)
an/o (anus)
aponeur/o (aponeurosis)
appendic/o (appendix)
arche/o (beginning)
arteri/o (artery)
athero/o (fatty plaque)
atri/o (atrium)
aur/I (ear)
aur/o (ear)
aut/o (self)
azot/o (nitrogen)
bacteri/o (bacteria)
balan/o (glans penis)

bi/o (life)
blast/o (developing cell)
blephar/o (eyelid)
bronch/I (bronchus)
bronch/o (bronchus)
burs/o (bursa)
calc/I (calcium)
cancer/o (cancer)
carcin/o (cancer)
cardi/o (heart)
carp/o (carpals)
caud/o (tail)
cec/o (cecum)
celi/o (abdomen)
cephal/o (head)
cerebell/o (cerebellum)
cerebr/o (cerebrum)
cervic/o (cervix)
cheil/o (lip)
cholangi/o (bile duct)
chol/e (gall)
chondro/o (cartilage)
chori/o (chorion)
chrom/o (color)
clavic/o (clavicle)

- 8 -

Common medical terminology *word roots* continued:

clavicul/o (clavicle)
col/o (colon)
colp/o (vagina)
core/o (pupil)
corne/o (cornea)
coron/o (heart)
cortic/o (cortex)
cor/o (pupil)
cost/o (rib)
crani/o (cranium)
cry/o (cold)
cutane/o (skin)
cyan/o (blue)
cyes/I (pregnancy)
cyst/o (bladder)
cyt/o (cell)
dacry/o (tear)
dermat/o (skin)
derm/o (skin)
diaphragmat/o(diaphragm)
dipl/o (double)
dips/o (thirst)
disk/o (disk)
dist/o (distal)
diverticul/o (diverticulum)
dors/o (back)
duoden/o (duodenum)
dur/o (dura)
ech/o (sound)
electr/o (electricity)
embry/o (embryo)
encephal/o (brain)
endocrin/o (endocrine)
enter/o (intestine)
epididym/o (epididymis)
epiglott/o (epiglottis)
episi/o (vulva)
epitheli/o (epithelium)
erythr/o (red)
esophag/o (esophagus)
esthesi/o (sensation)
eti/o (cause of disease)
femor/o (femur)
fet/I (fetus)
fet/o (fetus)
fibr/o (fibrous tissue)
fibul/o (fibula)

gangli/o (ganglion)
ganglion/o (ganglion)
gastr/o (stomach)
gingiv/o (gum)
glomerul/o (glomerulus)
gloss/o (tongue)
glyc/o (sugar)
gnos/o (knowledge)
gravid/o (pregnancy)
gynec/o (woman)
gyn/o (woman)
hem/o (blood)
hemat/o (blood)
hepat/o (liver)
herni/o (hernia)
heter/o (other)
hidr/o (sweat)
hist/o (tissue)
humer/o (humerus)
hydr/o (water)
hymen/o (hymen)
hyster/o (uterus)
ile/o (ileum)
ili/o (ilium)
infer/o (inferior)
irid/o (iris)
iri/o (iris)
ischi/o (ischium)
ischo/o (blockage)
jejun/o (jejunum)
kal/I (potassium)
kary/o (nucleus)
kerat/o (hard)
kinesi/o (motion)
kyph/o (hump)
lacrim/o (tear duct)
lact/o (milk)
lamin/o (lamina)
lapar/o (abdomen)
laryng/o (larynx)
later/o (lateral)
lei/o (smooth)
leuk/o (white)
lingu/o (tongue)
lip/o (fat)
lith/o (stone)
lord/o (flexed forward)
lumb/o (lumbar)
lymph/o (lymph)
mamm/o (breast)

- 9 -

Common medical terminology *word roots*
continued:

mandibul/o (mandible)
mast/o (breast)
mastoid/o (mastoid)
maxill/o (maxilla)
meat/o (opening)
melan/o (black)
mening/o (meninges)
menisc/o (meniscus)
men/o (menstruation)
ment/o (mind)
metr/I (uterus)
metr/o (uterus)
mon/o (one)
muc/o (mucus)
myc/o (fungus)
myel/o (spinal cord)
myelon/o (bone marrow)
myos/o (muscle)
my/o (muscle)
nas/o (nose)
nat/o (birth)
necr/o (death)
nephr/o (kidney)
neur/o (nerve)
noct/I (night)
ocul/o (eye)
olig/o (few)
omphal/o (navel)
onc/o (tumor)
onych/o (nail)
oophor/o (ovary)
ophthalm/o (eye)
opt/o (vision)
orchid/o (testicle)
orch/o (testicle)
organ/o (organ)
or/o (mouth)
orth/o (straight)
oste/o (bone)
ot/o (ear)
ox/I (oxygen)
pachy/o (thick)
palat/o (palate)
pancreat/o (pancreas)
parathyroid/o (parathyroid gland)
par/o (labor)
patell/o (patella)

path/o (disease)
pelv/I (pelvis)
perine/o (peritoneum)
petr/o (stone)
phalang/o (pharynx)
phas/o (speech)
phleb/o (vein)
phot/o (light)
phren/o (mind)
plasm/o (plasma)
pleur/o (pleura)
pneumat/o (lung)
pneum/o (lung)
pneumon/o (lung)
poli/o (gray matter)
polyp/o (small growth)
poster/o (posterior)
prim/I (first)
proct/o (rectum)
prostat/o (prostate gland)
proxim/o (proximal)
pseud/o (fake)
psych/o (mind)
pub/o (pubis)
puerper/o (childbirth)
pulmon/o (lung)
pupill/o (pupil)
pyel/o (renal pelvis)
pylor/o (pylorus)
py/o (pus)
quadr/I (four)
rachi/o (spinal)
radic/o (nerve)
radicul/o (nerve)
radi/o (radius)
rect/o (rectum)
ren/o (kidney)
retin/o (retina)
rhabd/o (striated)
rhin/o (nose)
rhytid/o (wrinkles)
rhiz/o (nerve)
salping/o (fallopian tube)
sacr/o (sacrum)
scapul/o (scapula)
scler/o (sclera)
scoli/o (curved)
seb/o (sebum)
sept/o (septum)
sial/o (saliva)

Common medical terminology *word roots* continued:

sinus/o (sinus)
somat/o (body)
son/o (sound)
spermat/o (sperm)
sphygm/o (pulse)
spir/o (breathe)
splen/o (spleen)
spondyl/o (vertebra)
staped/o (stapes)
staphyl/o (clusters)
stern/o (sternum)
steth/o (chest)
stomat/o (mouth)
strept/o (chain-like)
super/o (superior)
synovi/o (synovia)
system/o (system)
tars/o (tarsal)
tendin/o (tendon)
ten/o (tendon)
test/o (testicle)
therm/o (heat)
thorac/o (thorax)
thromb/o (clot)
thym/o (thymus)
thyroid/o (thyroid gland)
thyr/o (thyroid gland)

tibi/o (tibia)
tom/o (pressure)
tonsill/o (tonsils)
toxic/o (poison)
trachel/o (trachea)
trich/o (hair)
tympan/o (eardrum)
uln/o (ulna)
ungu/o (nail)
ureter/o (ureter)
urethr/o (urethra)
urin/o (urine)
ur/o (urine)
uter/o (uterus)
uvul/o (uvula)
vagin/o (vagina)
valv/o (valve)
valvul/o (valve)
vas/o (vessel)
ven/o (vein)
ventricul/o (ventricle)
ventro/o (frontal)
vertebr/o (vertebra)
vesic/o (bladder)
vesicul/o (seminal vesicles)
viscer/o (internal organs)
vulv/o (vulva)
xanth/o (yellow)
xer/o (dry)

Standardized terminology and abbreviations

Standardized terminology and abbreviations are vital for patient safety. Use abbreviations to save time and space *only when there is no potential for confusion over the meaning of your message.* Avoid Latin if there is an accepted English equivalency. Your Medical Records manager decides acceptable terminology and forbidden abbreviations. If you work in a small office and are in charge of Medical Records, use the list of safe terms from The American Society for Testing and Materials' (ASTM) and the list of dangerous abbreviations from the Institute for Safe Medication Practices (ISMP). The Joint Commission on Accreditation of Healthcare Organizations (JCAHO) also has a "Do Not Use" List for medical abbreviations and symbols that are included on the ISMP's more comprehensive list. Post them throughout your office. Use one type of units only. For example, do not use SI units (International System of Measurement) for Lab and Imperial units for Pharmacy without listing equivalencies. Adopt the U.S. Postal Service database's two-letter abbreviations for states.

Health professionals use abbreviations to save time when charting or to be discreet when speaking around a patient. Abbreviations take these forms:

- Brief form means shortening a common term or difficult to pronounce term, for example: "telephone" into "phone" and "Papanicolaou smear" into "Pap smear"
- Acronym means making word out of a phrase, for example: laser stands for light amplification by stimulated emission of radiation
- Initialism means making a word from the first letters of words in a phrase, and pronouncing the series of letters, for example, MRI for magnetic resonance imaging or HIV for human immunodeficiency virus.
- Eponym means naming a test or sign for its discoverer, for example, Coomb's test and McBurney's sign

Potentially lethal abbreviations to avoid are:
- Homonyms — Same pronunciation but different meaning, such as ileum and ilium
- Synonyms — Different words with similar meanings, such as dead and deceased

Medical abbreviations and acronyms
AIDS: acquired immunodeficiency syndrome
A.D.: right ear, auris dextra (* on ISMP's list of error prone abbreviations)
A.S.: left ear, auris sinistra (* on ISMP's list of error prone abbreviations)
A.U.: both ears, auris utraque (* on ISMP's list of error prone abbreviations)
O.D.: right eye, oculus dexter (* on ISMP's list of error prone abbreviations)
O.S.: left eye, oculus sinister (* on ISMP's list of error prone abbreviations)
O.U.: both eyes, oculus uterque (* on ISMP's list of error prone abbreviations)
CA: cancer or carcinoma
CBC and diff: complete blood count and differential
CHF: congestive heart failure
TAHBSO: complete hysterectomy; total abdominal hysterectomy, bilateral salpingo-oophorectomy
CABG: (pronounced "cabbage") coronary artery bypass graft
DNR : do not resuscitate. No codes should be called for this patient and no heroic measures should be taken to revive patient if the patient stops breathing.
DTR: deep tendon reflexes
D&C: dilatation and curettage, used to cure uterine bleeding or for early abortion
ECG or ECG: electrocardiogram
ELISA: enzyme-linked immunosorbent assay, used to test for antibodies and antigens
Fabere: flexion-abduction-external rotation-extension test, part of a physical to measure the patient's range of motion
HPI: history of present illness
Laser: light amplification by stimulated emission of radiation, a tool to carve tissue
P&A: percussion and auscultation, as in, "The lungs were clear to P&A."
PVH: persistent viral hepatitis
PND: postnasal drainage (can also mean paroxysmal nocturnal dyspnea in a sleep study)
simkin: simulation kinetics analysis
p.c.: after meals
a.c.: before meals
h.s.: bedtime
OD: daily [NOTE: Do not confuse with o.d., right eye.] (* on ISMP's list of error prone abbreviations)
ad lib: freely or whenever desired
p.r.n.: as needed

with: cum or letter c with macron
without: sine or letter s with a flat macron line on top
cm: centimeters
cc: cubic centimeters
gtt: drops
g: grams
kg: kilograms
q.4h.: every four hours
mEq: milliequivalents

Common abbreviations
Autonomic nervous system - ANS
Anterior - ant
As soon as possible - ASAP
Arteriovenous - AV
Twice a day - bid
Blood pressure - BP
Beats per minute – bpm
Blood urea nitrogen- BUN
Biopsy- Bx
Culture and sensitivity – C&S
Calcium - Ca
Completer blood count - CBC
Colony count - CC
Carcinoma embryonic antigen - CEA
Chloride - Cl
Central nervous system - CNS
Creatine phosphokinase   - CPK
Cardiopulmonary resuscitation - CPR
Cerebrospinal fluid - CSF
Cardiovascular - CV
Central venous pressure - CVP
Discharge – D/C
Distilled water - DW
Diagnosis - Dx
Estimated blood loss - EBL
In the manner prescribed – e.m.p.
Estrogen replacement therapy - ERT
Erythrocyte sedimentation rate - ESR
Etiology - etiol
Fasting blood sugar - FBS
Iron - Fe
Follicle-stimulating hormone - FSH
Gram - g
Gastroesophageal reflux disease - GERD
Gradually – Grad.
Glucose tolerance test - GTT
Hour - h
Hypodermic- H or hypo.
Hemodialysis- HD

- 13 -

Hemoglobin and hematocrit - H&H
Hematocrit- Hct
Mercury- Hg
Hemoglobin- Hgb
Human immunodeficiency virus- HIV
History and physical – H&P
Intramuscular- IM
Intravenous- IV
Potassium - K
Potassium Chloride - KCL
Keep Vein Open - KVO
Laboratory – lab
Medications – meds.
Multiple Sclerosis – MS
Sodium – Na
Newborn – NB
Negative – neg
NPO – nothing by mouth
Oxygen – O_2
Overdose – OD
After meals - pc
Packed Cell Volume – PCV
Between noon and midnight – PM
Positive – pos.
Postoperatively – post-op
Packed Red Blood Cells – PRBC
Prostatic specific antigen – PSA
Prothrombin time – PT
Physical Therapy – PT
Every day – qd
Every other day – qod
Immediately – stat
Three times a day - tid

Pluralizing medical terms

Most medical laboratory terms derive from Latin and Greek. Most Latinate terms originated from the Greek. The basic rules for pluralizing medical terms are as follows:

Rule	Example
a changes to –ata	Stigma to stigmata Condyloma to condylomata
-on changes to -a	Criterion to criteria Phenomenon to phenomena
-s changes to –des	Iris to irides Arthritis to arthritides
Feminine a ending changes to ae	Ulna to ulnae Concha to conchae
Masculine ending us changes to i	Radius to radii Musculus to musculi

Rule	Example
Neuter ending um changes to a	Bacteri*um* to bacteri*a* Trepone*um* to Trepone*a*
-osis changes to -oses	Diagn*osis* to diagn*oses* Anastom*osis* to anastom*oses*
-x changes to –ces or –ges	Phalan*x* to phalan*ges* Vari*x* to vari*ces*

Medical and surgical specialties

The suffix *-ology* means "the study of", and the suffix –iatrics means "medical treatment". Add the body system root to obtain the name of the specialty:

- Anesthesiology — Study of pain relief
- Bariatrics — Treatment of obesity
- Cardiology — Study of the heart
- Dermatology — Study of the skin
- Endocrinology — Study of the hormone system
- Gastroenterology — Study of the digestive system
- Geriatrics —Treatment of the elderly
- Hematology — Study of the blood
- Neurology — Study of the nervous system
- Obstetrics — Treatment of pregnant women
- Pediatrics — Treatment of children
- Psychiatry — Treatment of the mind
- Radiology —Study of radiation (for medical imaging)
- Rheumatology — Study of rheumatoid diseases, like arthritis
- Toxicology — Study of poisons
- Urology — Study of the urinary system

Terms in doctor's notes

b.i.d.: twice a day

t.i.d: three times a day

q.i.d.: four times a day (* on ISMP's list of error prone abbreviations)

I.M.: within the muscle, intramuscular

I.V.: within the vein, intravenous

p.o.: by mouth

Rx: Recipe for the prescription literally means "Take thou". Also called superscription.

Sig: Write on the label for the patient. Also called signature.

STAT: immediately

NPO: Nihil per os (nothing by mouth), a routine precaution before surgery to prevent aspiration of vomitus.

Auscultation: Listening to organ sounds to make a diagnosis. Immediate auscultation uses only the ear. Mediate auscultation is with a stethoscope.

Diagnosis: When the doctor names or identifies the disease, judging by its signs and symptoms.

Palpation: Touching with the hands over the patient's skin to determine the size and consistency of underlying organs to help make the diagnosis, e.g., enlarged lymph glands, hot abdomen.

Percussion: Tapping the skin over an organ to determine its condition by the sound it makes.

Reference sources for medical terminology

Reliable reference sources to check correct spelling, selection and use of medical terminology are listed below:

- Abbreviations: Use safe terms and definitions from The American Society for Testing and Materials' (ASTM). Obtain a list of dangerous abbreviations to be avoided from the Institute for Safe Medication Practices.
- Style guides: Provide guidelines for format and presentation in documents. Use the *American Medical Association Manual of Style: A Guide for Authors and Editors* for an overview.
- Anatomy and physiology texts: Contain essential information regarding body structure, function of body parts, disease processes, and common health disorders. *Grey's Anatomy* is the classic.
- Specialty texts: When you need help with specialty transcriptions, try Sloan's *Medical Word Book*, Tessier's *Surgical Word Book*, and Pagana's *Laboratory and Diagnostic Tests*.
- English dictionary: Helps with spelling, definitions, and pronunciation. *Cambridge Dictionary of American English* is the standard.

Ethical and Legal Issues

Scope of practice

Scope of practice is a list of tasks that a patient care technician is allowed to perform as determined by the state certification board. It is the responsibility of the patient care technician to be aware of what tasks she can and cannot perform. Any activity that does not appear on the list falls outside the patient care technician's scope of practice; if the patient care technician is caught performing an activity that is not on the list, she runs the risk of losing her certification. The patient care technician is liable for any harm that comes to the patient as a result of the patient care technician performing an activity that is outside her scope of practice.

Tasks not part of scope of practice

There are a number of tasks that fall outside the patient care technician's scope of practice. A patient care technician is not allowed to receive orders from a doctor; only a nurse can write orders. A patient care technician may not insert or remove devices from a patient's body, such as indwelling catheters, IVs, or rectal tubes. Also, a patient care technician may not perform any sort of sterile procedure. In most cases, a patient care technician may not administer medications. Some states allow a patient care technician to assist the patient in self-administration of medication under specific circumstances. The patient care technician may only assist in medication administration if she receives special training and may only assist in administering certain medications.

If a patient care technician feels she is being asked to perform an assignment that is outside of her scope of practice, she should talk to the charge nurse privately after the assignments have been given. The patient care technician should explain why she feels uncomfortable about the assignment. If necessary, the facility's policy and procedure manual can be consulted to confirm if the assigned task falls within the patient care technician's scope of practice. If it does, and the patient care technician still feels uncomfortable, she should request that the charge nurse be present while the task is being performed to ensure it is performed correctly.

Refusing assignments

A patient care technician must have a valid reason to refuse an assignment. There are a number of reasons why she might do so. A particular assignment might not be part of a patient care technician's scope of practice. The patient care technician might feel uncomfortable with the assignment as a result of not knowing how to perform a task or may feel it is unethical or illegal. The patient care technician may refuse an assignment if she feels performing the task will cause harm to the patient or may place herself in danger if she were to perform that task.

Rights of delegation

It is important for a patient care technician to understand how a task is delegated in order to know if it is being delegated appropriately. The five rights of delegation can be utilized to determine if the assignment is appropriate. The first right refers to the task: whether the task can be delegated to another person or if it is more appropriate for it to be performed by the nurse. The second right refers to the circumstance; the patient care technician should ask herself if the patient is stable enough for the task to be safely performed. The third right refers to the right person. The patient care technician should ask herself if she feels she is able to perform the task appropriately. The fourth right refers to directions. The patient care technician should ask herself if she received adequate instructions regarding the assignment. The final right refers to supervision. The patient care technician should ask herself if she is going to have an appropriate amount of supervision while performing the task.

Delegation

Delegation refers to assigning a task to another person. It is within the nurse's scope of practice to assign tasks to the patient care technician; however, it is not within the patient care technician's scope of practice to assign tasks to others. Though the patient care technician is responsible for performing the task, it is the responsibility of the nurse to make sure that it is done properly and in a timely manner. When assigned a task, the patient care technician should make sure she understands how to perform that task. If she does not know how to do it, the patient care technician should either ask for instructions in order to perform the task safely or decline the assignment.

ADA and CLIA

Americans with Disabilities Act (ADA) of 1990:
- Prevents discrimination in employment
- Ensures access to public services, accommodations, and goods
- Provides sophisticated telecommunication services to facilitate the hearing and speech impaired.
- Requires medical offices to have ramps, entryways, and at least one treatment room that provides access and accommodates the needs of the disabled
- Applies to facilities with more than 15 employees, but all medical offices should strive to comply with ADA

Clinical Laboratory Improvement Amendment (CLIA) of 1988:
- Private research labs are exempt
- All other laboratories are controlled by the Centers for Medicare and Medicaid (CMS) and must:
- Be certified or licensed by an authorized accrediting body or the state
- Participate in proficiency testing and quality control, including positive and negative controls
- Have written procedures and policies, and requirements for monitoring, assessing, and correcting pre-and post-analytical problems
- Retain patient samples and records for specified times
- Toxicology tests require a CLIA number for data forwarding

OSHA and FDA

The U.S. Department of Labor's Occupational Safety and Health Administration (OSHA) sets standards for:
- Proper hand washing
- Wearing gloves and other personal protective equipment (PPE)
- Bagging specimens in biohazard bags
- Disposing of needles and lancets in a sharps safe
- Cleaning up spills to prevent spread of bloodborne pathogens
- Harmful chemical control
- Safe equipment use
- Adequate work space

You must check for updates regularly at OSHA's Web site at http://www.osha.gov and are required to adopt them as part of your standards of practice.

The U.S. Food & Drug Administration (FDA):
- Assigns the official (generic) name for drugs when it approves them
- Reports recalls and adverse events through *MedWatch*
- Publishes a free, downloadable *Orange Book* of approved drugs at http://www.accessdata.fda.gov/scripts/cder/ob/default.cfm
- Divides drugs into five schedules, based on their potential for abuse, numbered Schedule I (illegal) to Schedule V(benign)
- Sets the temperature regulations for dish sanitization

Medical jurisprudence, contracts, torts, and criminal laws

Jurisprudence is the legal system set up and enforced at various governmental levels. Civil and criminal laws that pertain to medical situations are medical jurisprudence. Medical jurisprudence also involves applying the science of medicine to legal issues such as forensics or paternity testing. Civil laws are more often invoked in the medical setting, as they pertain to either contracts or torts. A contract is an enforceable covenant between two or more competent individuals. An agreement between a doctor and his or her patient is a contract. It can be an *expressed* contract, with written or verbal terms, or it can be an *implied* contract, where actions create the contract. Tort law governs the other branch of civil law. Torts relate to standards of care and wrongful actions that cause injury to a patient. Criminal laws speak to crimes that endanger society in general. There are occasions when criminal law may apply to medicine, usually resulting in fines, incarceration, and discipline by the state medical board.

Contract law

There is an expressed or an implied contract between the doctor and patient. The medical assistant and other personnel are the doctor's agents. The doctor is ultimately responsible for breach of contract under the *Doctrine of Respondeat Superior*. Nevertheless, the assistant's words or actions regarding care are legally binding upon the doctor. Breach of contract is failure to fulfill and complete the terms of the contract. There are four situations where a contract can be legally abandoned:

- The patient releases the doctor by failure to return for treatment; ideally, the patient sends the doctor a certified letter of discharge, but this is not required
- The patient/guardian does not comply with specific instructions from the doctor regarding care
- The patient no longer requires treatment
- The doctor formally withdraws from the case by sending a certified letter to the patient explaining the situation, to preclude any charges of patient abandonment

Patient consents

The types of patient consents needed to do a procedure are as follows:
- Informed Consent - a competent person gives voluntary permission for a medical procedure after receiving adequate information about the risk of, methods used and consequences of the procedure
- Expressed Consent - permission given by patient verbally or in writing for a procedure
- Implied Consent - the patient's actions gives permission for the procedure without verbal or written consent for example going to the emergency room or holding out arm when told need to draw blood.
- HIV Consent - special permission given to administer a test for detecting the human immunodeficiency virus.
- Parental Consent for Minors - a parent or a legal guardian must give permission for procedures administered to underage patients depending on the state law may range from 18 to 21 years old.

Informed consent
Informed consent protects patients by ensuring they or those legally responsible for them are fully educated about tests, treatments, and procedures. The patient has the legal right to know about his/her own condition. The exceptions are life-threatening emergencies and legal incompetence. Informed consent protects healthcare professionals from battery lawsuits. Informed consent is obtained when the patient is given written information in regards to the treatment plan, risks, benefits, and alternative treatment options, the provider truthfully answers any questions, and the patient/parent/guardian comprehends the discussion. The patient or legal guardian then *voluntarily* signs the consent form, without duress or coercion. You must obtain signed consent from the parent/guardian before treatment commences. Moreover, it is advisable to obtain the minor patient's assent prior to the procedure. Always keep the original informed consent form in the patient's chart. Assent should also be recorded in the medical record.

Patient rights

Patient's Bill of Rights
The Patient's Bill of Rights is a list of rights that the patient can expect to receive while he stays in a hospital or an extended-care facility. This list of rights may differ in wording from hospital to hospital but generally contains similar provisions. The Bill of Rights is typically accompanied by a list of responsibilities that the patient should adhere to in order to ensure his treatment is effective. It is important that the patient be made aware of his rights and responsibilities as soon after admission as possible.

Right of confidentiality

The patient has the right to have his case discussed only by those who are directly responsible for his care. Unless a patient care technician is caring for the patient, she should not review his chart or discuss his case. Furthermore, once the patient care technician is no longer providing care to the patient, she should not access his records. After the patient is transferred to another unit of the hospital, the patient care technician should not access his files. Patient information should be discussed in areas where other people cannot overhear it to prevent laypeople from hearing details about the patient's care.

Right of privacy

Patients have a right to personal privacy. The patient care technician should make an effort to protect the patient's privacy by maintaining his dignity during patient care procedures. While bathing the patient or taking him off of the bedpan, the curtain or door to the room should be closed to prevent other people from seeing in. The patient's right to privacy also applies to his health information. Details of the patient's case should only be discussed with the family members that the patient specifies. Many facilities have developed a system involving a privacy code number that is only given to the family members that are to receive information regarding the patient. Unless the family member is able to provide the privacy code number, the patient care technician can only confirm the patient's presence on the unit.

Right of informed consent

The idea of informed consent originally came about in reference to experimental treatment. However, it has come to encompass the type of information that should be provided prior to every test, procedure, or treatment. Before signing the consent form, the patient has the right to be informed about all of the risks and benefits involved in the proposed treatment, as well as the risks and benefits involved in refusing the treatment. He should be told which doctors will be involved in his care and what medications he will receive. The doctor should provide this information prior to the procedure, either directly to the patient or to the patient's health care power of attorney.

Right of respectful care

When a patient enters the hospital, he has the right to be treated respectfully by those who are providing care to him. The patient cannot be discriminated against because of age, gender, race, or religion. He also cannot be denied treatment as a result of the circumstances surrounding his hospitalization. For example, the patient cannot be denied care for injuries acquired during the commission of a crime. While the patient is in the hospital, he has the right to expect care to be provided safely by competent staff. While the patient is in the hospital or extended-care facility, reasonable measures should be taken to accommodate the patient's cultural or religious requests, provided they do not interfere with the care of other patients.

Rights regarding telephone and mail

The patient has the right to have regular access to a telephone in order to communicate with family members. The patient should be informed as to where the telephone is located and how to use it. The patient should also have an expectation of privacy during his telephone conversations. The patient's conversations should not be monitored or recorded in any way. The patient has similar rights regarding the mail. Patient mail should not be opened without his consent, and any outgoing mail should be sent without being read by members of the health care staff.

Freedom of choice

The patient's right to freedom of choice works in conjunction with the right of informed consent. Once he has been provided the necessary information, the patient has the right to choose what treatments he will receive. He is free to make this decision without pressure from the health care staff. Once he has made his decision, it cannot be undermined unless he makes the decision to change treatments. Conversely, if the patient decides to stop the treatment, he may do so, though the doctor should remind the patient about the risks and benefits involved in quitting the treatment.

DNR order

A Do Not Resuscitate (DNR) order outlines the type of heroic measures that may be undertaken if the patient's heart or breathing were to stop during the course of treatment. The DNR order typically specifies if the patient desires emergent intubation, CPR, or defibrillation. The doctor typically writes a DNR order after an extensive conversation with the patient about his wishes regarding his care. In some cases, the patient may choose to have some of the emergency treatments, but not all of them. It is important for the patient care technician to familiarize herself with the types of emergency treatment the patient wants. The patient can reverse a DNR at any time. If the patient verbalizes a desire to change his code status, the charge nurse should be notified.

Medical durable power of attorney

A medical durable power of attorney designates a specific person to make any medically related decisions if the patient should become unable to make the decisions himself. Durable power of attorney would take effect if the patient were to become confused or comatose. The durable power of attorney is typically filed by a lawyer prior to hospitalization. The person who has been made medical power of attorney should make an effort to learn the patient's wishes regarding health care decisions. If the patient becomes hospitalized, the family should present the durable power of attorney paperwork as soon as possible. If the patient's family brings in a copy of the patient's durable power of attorney, the patient care technician should inform the nurse immediately.

Advanced directives

Advanced directives detail the patient's wishes regarding end-of-life care. They address whether the patient wants to receive long-term mechanical ventilation, continuous dialysis, or nourishment via a feeding tube. The advanced directives may also address whether the patient wants to be an organ or tissue donor after death. The patient typically sees a lawyer to have his advanced directives prepared prior to hospitalization. Health care providers should be made aware immediately upon hospitalization if the patient has advanced directives. If the patient's family brings in a copy of the patient's advanced directives, the patient care technician should notify the nurse immediately.

Experimental treatment

The patient has very specific rights when it comes to experimental treatment. Like any other procedure, informed consent is required prior to beginning treatment. The patient should be notified of the experimental nature of the treatment, as well as any potential risks and benefits involved in accepting the treatment. The patient should be approached in a manner that is not threatening. If the patient refuses the treatment, he has the right to be informed of other treatments that may be performed in place of the experimental treatment. Care cannot be refused to the patient based upon refusal of an experimental treatment.

Right to continuity of care

Continuity of care is defined as high-quality health care provided continuously and consistently. Often, continuity of care can be difficult to achieve in a health care setting because of the number of practitioners that can get involved in a patient's case. Continuity of care may break down for a number of reasons, including a doctor's lack of familiarity with a treatment plan or lack of communication among the health care team. In order to maintain continuity of care, there should be frequent conferences between the health care team and the patient to ensure that everyone is in agreement regarding the plan of care.

Right of refusal

If the patient is alert and oriented, he has the right to refuse any treatment or procedure. This includes simple procedures, such as turning or a bath. If the patient decides, for example, that he does not want to be turned, he should not be scolded or coerced for his decision. He should be informed of the risks involved in not being turned. If the patient continues to refuse, then the patient care technician should not argue. The charge nurse should be notified so that the proper documentation can be made. If possible, the patient care technician may offer the procedure again at a later time.

Money and valuables

Though it is unwise to bring a large sum of money or valuables to a hospital setting, it is sometimes unavoidable. Dentures and hearing aids, for example, are very costly pieces of equipment, but they are also necessary for everyday use. If the patient enters the hospital with money or valuables, he has the right to expect that the hospital will take reasonable steps to protect his property. The patient has the right to maintain his own accounts when he enters a long-term care facility. At no point should a member of the health care facility access the patient's financial accounts. If the patient is unable to take responsibility for his financial matters, the social worker should be contacted to make necessary arrangements.

Right to identification of health care workers

The patient has the right to know the names of the people that are providing care for him. On a given day, the patient may encounter a number of people, including doctors, nurses, physical therapists, and patient care technicians. A name badge clearly identifies a person as an employee of the health care facility and states the individual's position. It informs the patient of what to expect from the employee. When a patient care technician enters the patient's room, she should wear her nametag above the waist in a location that is clearly visible. She should also identify herself in order to prevent confusion.

Rights of a dying patient

A patient's rights should be closely respected at all times, especially when he is dying. Every effort should be made to place the patient in a private room. When the family is present, the door to the room should be closed; if the door cannot be closed, then the curtain should be pulled shut. Reports regarding the patient should be given where others cannot overhear. Any monitor alarms should be turned off or silenced. Privacy should be respected if the patient needs to be cleaned up and during postmortem care. When transporting the body to the morgue, the morgue cart should be kept covered to protect the patient's identity.

<u>Rights of patients with disabilities</u>

Every effort should be taken to protect the rights of patients with disabilities. If the patient is hearing or visually impaired, the health care team should tailor its communication techniques to make sure the patient understands what is being said to him. If the patient is confused or mentally challenged, the patient's health care proxy must be kept informed of his status and conferred with regarding aspects of his care. If the patient does not have a health care proxy and there is no family available, a temporary proxy can be named to act in the patient's best interests until the patient is well enough to do so himself. If necessary, the health care facility's social work team should be notified to aid in protecting the rights of a patient with disabilities.

Protecting patient valuables

If the patient comes into the hospital with large sums of money or jewelry, the patient should be encouraged to give it to a family member to take home. If a family member is not present, permission should be obtained from the patient to put the valuables in the hospital safe. If the patient consents, security should be called, the items catalogued, and a receipt given to the patient. If the patient is unconscious or comatose, the valuables should be locked up until he is able to give consent. If the patient has a valuable that is required for daily use, such as glasses, hearing aids, or dentures, every effort must be taken to protect these items. The patient should be provided a case marked with his name on it. When the items are not in use, they should be kept close at hand in a place where they are not at risk for breaking or being lost.

Liability

Liability refers to the responsibility of a person to act within the confines of the law. In the eyes of the law, a person must take responsibility for his own actions. If a patient care technician fails to perform a task to the best of her ability and harm comes to the patient, she can be considered liable. Similarly, if the patient care technician performs a task that falls outside of her scope of practice and harm comes to the patient, she is considered liable. In order to maintain safe practice, it is important for a patient care technician to perform tasks exactly as she learned them, without taking shortcuts. She should also make an effort to keep her skills and knowledge up to date with current health care trends.

Assault

Assault refers to the threat or attempt to touch or inflict physical harm on another person. The threat could be verbal or physical, such as a threatening gesture or advancing toward a person in a threatening way. Caution must be taken while caring for a patient; if the patient refuses a treatment and the patient care technician attempts to force the patient to receive the treatment, she may be liable for assault. It is important to remember that the patient does not have to be harmed in order for the patient care technician to be found liable for assault. It is only necessary to prove that the patient felt threatened in a particular situation.

Tort

A tort is a wrong that is committed in a civil case. There are two types of torts: unintentional and intentional. In an unintentional tort, a person commits a wrong against another person without intending to cause harm. For example, if a patient care technician forgets to put the side rails back up on the bed and the patient falls and injures himself as a result, that could be considered an unintentional tort. An intentional tort occurs when a person has the intention of causing harm to another person. An example of an intentional tort is if the patient care technician leaves the unit without telling anybody, and the patient becomes injured while he is not being monitored.

Negligence

Negligence is the failure to perform care in the manner in which that person was trained. A patient care technician can be charged with negligence if she does not act in a way that is reasonable for a person with her level of training. For example, if the patient care technician leaves a patient unattended in the shower and the patient falls and injures himself, the patient care technician could be found negligent. A patient care technician can avoid being accused of negligence by performing procedures exactly as she learned how to do them, without taking shortcuts. If the patient care technician is unsure how to perform a procedure, she should not hesitate to ask for assistance.

The patient care technician should be observant for any signs of negligence in the health care facility. Negligence can include failing to perform important tasks, such as turning or ambulating, or performing patient care activities in a manner that is unsafe. If the patient care technician sees another member of the health care team behaving in a way that is negligent, she should report that behavior to the charge nurse. If it is the charge nurse who is behaving negligently, the patient care technician should utilize the proper chain of command to make sure the behavior is addressed. She should not try to confront the negligent coworker herself.

Battery

Battery refers to the act of touching a person without permission. It could refer to a violent act or an unintended act. A patient care technician might also be accused of battery for performing a procedure on a patient without his consent. In order to protect herself from being accused of battery, a patient care technician should take a moment to explain the procedure to the patient prior to beginning and obtain consent from the patient to perform the procedure. If the patient refuses the procedure, the patient care technician should try to explain the reasons why the procedure is necessary but should not attempt to force the patient to have the procedure performed.

Defamation

When a person makes statements about another person that causes damage to the individual's reputation, she can be accused of defamation. Slander refers to spoken defamation. For example, if a patient care technician spreads rumors that a patient has HIV, that patient care technician can be accused of slander. Libel refers to a written statement that causes injury to another person's reputation. For example, if the patient care technician writes an article that a doctor is practicing without appropriate licensure and that article is untrue, she can be accused of libel. A patient care technician can avoid being accused of slander by avoiding saying negative things about other people. By spreading rumors, the patient care technician is acting unprofessionally and places herself at risk for being accused of defamation.

Invasion of privacy

The patient has a right to keep details about himself private. Invasion of privacy refers to failure to maintain the patient's right to privacy by relaying personal information without the patient's consent. The patient's privacy can be invaded if the patient care technician shares details about the patient's health history with others or by inadvertently leaving sensitive documents where others can easily see them. A patient care technician can avoid being accused of invasion of privacy by only discussing details of the case with those who are directly involved in the care of the patient. If a person who is not part of the patient's immediate family wants information regarding the patient's treatment, the patient care technician should refer him to the charge nurse.

Malpractice

Malpractice is a type of negligence that is committed by a professional who needs to maintain a license in order to practice. In a case of malpractice, a professional fails to act according to standards of care within her profession, which results in harm coming to the patient. Malpractice is more severe than negligence; it takes into account the professional's higher level of training when considering the wrong that was committed by the health care professional. Patient care technicians cannot be sued for malpractice as they are only required to maintain certification. However, they can still be sued for negligence.

Fraud

When a person commits fraud, she deliberately misrepresents herself for personal gain. It can be considered a violation of either civil or criminal law. A patient care technician would commit fraud if she claimed to be a nurse or a doctor in the presence of a patient. It is also considered fraud to lie about one's qualifications or certifications on a resume in order to secure a job. A patient care technician can avoid being accused of fraud by clearly identifying herself when dealing with a patient. She can also avoid being accused of fraud by acting within her scope of practice.

Abandonment

Abandonment occurs when a patient care technician leaves without notifying others or securing another person to provide care in her place. If harm befalls a patient while the patient care technician is absent of her duties, she can be accused of abandonment. A patient care technician can avoid being accused of abandonment by asking another patient care technician to cover her patients and informing the charge nurse prior to leaving the unit. She should also make an effort to make sure all of her patients are safe and secure prior to giving report and leaving the unit.

False imprisonment

False imprisonment refers to confining a person to an area against his will. It is typically used in reference to use of restraints. Restraints are an acceptable tool to be used as a last resort in order to protect both the patient and the safety of others. False imprisonment refers to the use of restraints without an order or in a situation in which it is inappropriate to restrain the patient. A patient could also be falsely imprisoned if he is confined to the health care facility when he wishes to leave. If the patient expresses a desire to leave the hospital and he is alert and able to make decisions for himself, the patient care technician should avoid attempting to force the patient to stay. Instead, she should notify the charge nurse or the supervisor immediately.

Theft

Theft is the removal of another person's money or belongings without his knowledge. A patient care technician is guilty of theft if she takes a patient's belongings, even if the stolen item is not being used or is not of significant monetary value. Though the health care facility takes steps to avoid hiring people who might steal from patients, the patient care technician should be vigilant as well. The patient care technician should try to avoid theft by not leaving the patient's belongings in plain sight when they are not in use. If she sees someone stealing a patient's belongings or acting suspiciously, she should report the behavior to the charge nurse immediately.

Abuse

Abuse is any sort of action that results in the physical harm, mental harm, or death of the patient. It is a criminal act and most typically results in imprisonment. Abusive actions can be deliberate or can be the result of negligence. It can take a number of forms, including physical, psychological, verbal, sexual, or financial abuse. Abuse can be subtle, and some victims of abuse may be reluctant to come forward. The patient care technician should be vigilant for any signs of abuse and report any findings to the charge nurse immediately.

Psychological abuse
Psychological or emotional abuse occurs when a person uses psychological attacks in order to intimidate or humiliate another person. It is typically done in order to coerce the person into doing something that he does not want to do. Psychological abuse can include teasing, threatening harm, or abandonment. Psychological abuse can be difficult to identify because it does not necessarily leave physical marks. A person who has been psychologically abused may show vague symptoms, such as chronic depression, anxiety, anger, or posttraumatic stress disorder. In many cases, other types of abuse accompany psychological abuse.

Verbal abuse
Verbal abuse refers to using words and threats in order to demean or upset another person. Verbal abuse includes threatening another person, raising one's voice in anger, or using profanity or derogatory statements toward the other person. It can be difficult to identify a person who is being verbally abused. They may complain of vague symptoms, such as depression, anxiety, anger, or a feeling of hopelessness. In many cases, the victim may blame himself or herself for the abuse or may be overcome with hopelessness that the abuse cannot be stopped. Verbal abuse is often accompanied by physical abuse.

Sexual abuse
Sexual abuse is any unwanted sexual behavior directed from one person to another. It includes any sexually suggestive comments or gestures, unwanted touching or fondling, or coercion to perform a sexual act. Additional forms of sexual abuse include sexual harassment or behavior that is sexually demeaning. Other forms of abuse may accompany sexual abuse in order to frighten the victim into maintaining silence.

Possible signs of sexual abuse include bruising around the perineal area, complaints of abdominal pain, or reoccurring yeast or urinary tract infections. The patient may also exhibit depression or increased anxiety or anger.

Physical abuse

Physical abuse is the most obvious form of abuse. It occurs when one person deliberately inflicts harm on another person and may be accompanied by verbal, emotional, or sexual abuse. Signs of physical abuse include bruising or abrasions with a distinctive shape, such as a fist or foot. Any injuries that do not coincide with the provided explanation should be suspected. For example, a caregiver states that the patient burned himself while cooking. The explanation would be suspect if the burns are in a suspicious place, such as on the inner arm or on the abdomen. If a caregiver refuses to leave the patient's side during an interview or insists upon speaking for the patient, this behavior should also be suspected.

Financial abuse

Financial abuse occurs when a person takes the money and belongings of another person. The elderly are most commonly the victims of financial abuse. Forms of financial abuse include forcing a person to sign over property, using monthly disability checks for items other than the elderly person's care, or forging another person's signature.
Being observant is the best way to catch financial abuse. It is possible that the patient is being abused financially if the patient lacks basic amenities, such as appropriate clothing or necessary personal items, (e.g. glasses or hearing aids) despite adequate financial assistance.

Reporting abuse

It is the obligation of the health care facility to report any incidences of abuse to the state in order to protect the victim and remove him from the situation. The patient care technician should be vigilant for any signs of abuse and should report any signs of abuse to the charge nurse. This includes any physical signs of abuse, any statements made by the patient regarding abuse, or any signs of neglect. Once the findings have been reported to the charge nurse, the health care team will determine if any abuse has taken place and notify the proper authorities. The patient care technician should not try to discuss the subject with the victim by herself, and she should not attempt to confront or accuse the abuser.

The physician and other health professionals must report to authorities:
- Gunshot wounds
- Possible terrorist incidents, especially if they involve the spread of disease
- Known or suspected abuse of a child, senior, or disabled person
- Sexual assault of a juvenile or disabled person
- Poisoning
- Wounds intentionally caused by knives and sharp objects
- Criminal violence, including domestic violence
- Client-specific information for the central cancer registry
- Specific contagious diseases determined by each state

The PCT must keep a written record of the patient's information that was disclosed to authorities.

HIPAA

Congress enacted the Health Insurance Portability and Accountability Act (HIPAA) in 1996 in order to ensure the privacy of patient health information. It requires each health care facility to prepare a list of policies and procedures in order to protect patient information. This includes limiting the ability to access patient information to only those who provide direct patient care. HIPAA also requires each health care facility to come up with technological safeguards to prevent the removal of patient information from hospital computer systems. If the hospital system violates the standards set forth by HIPAA, the hospital may be subject to severe fines and other penalties.

HIPAA stands for Health Insurance Portability and Accountability Act of 1996. HIPAA's Title I regulates healthcare accessibility, especially in the cases of job change and loss; Title II regulates patient privacy rights. HIPAA requires:
- Every patient's medical record must bear a Unique Identifier to prevent misidentification
- Patients must be given access to their protected health information (medical records) at any time, upon request
- Only *relevant* health information can be disclosed to *authorized* parties
- A record must be kept of *every* disclosure
- Every patient or the parents/guardian must receive a *Notice of Privacy Practices*, outlining how the protected health information will be used
- Physical access to protected health information must be limited (including electronic files via password protection or swipe cards, firewall, and SSL encryption)
- Retired electronic equipment must have all data records wiped clean

Professional behavior in a therapeutic relationship

Your patient shares confidential information with you, which makes the patient vulnerable. At the beginning of a therapeutic relationship, the PCT is responsible for establishing:
- Trust
- Clear, identifiable boundaries
- Mutual expectations
- Confidentiality ground rules

Respond to your patient's needs, but pursue the treatment objectives established by the doctor foremost. Demonstrate acceptance, humor, and compassion to the patient, but keep an appropriate emotional and physical distance. Limit your patient contact to assisting with medical procedures, bookings, and casual conversation. It is unprofessional conduct to date or befriend patients, or give them insider information. Remember: *Your primary purpose is therapeutic.* Stay alert for:
- Inappropriate emotions imposed on another person (transference and countertransference)
- Conflict of interest (using the relationship for personal gain)

At the end of your therapeutic relationship, arrange a monitoring schedule, so your patient is not lost to follow-up.

Inappropriate comments from patient

Some patients may attempt to use sexual innuendo jokingly or as a way to ease their own discomfort. However, such comments are considered to be harassment. Members of the health care staff have a right to work in an environment that is free of harassment. Some may try to diffuse the situation with a joke, but this approach is typically ineffective in halting the abusive behavior. If the patient begins making inappropriate comments, the patient care technician should immediately inform the patient that his comments are unacceptable and will not be tolerated. This should be stated firmly, but politely. If the patient continues the inappropriate behavior, the charge nurse should be notified.

Behaving in an ethical manner

Behaving in an ethical manner refers to doing what is right. In order to provide ethically appropriate care, the patient care technician should strive to consistently provide high-quality care for her patients. In order for a patient care technician to behave in an ethical manner, she must act in a manner that is in accordance with the standards of practice within her state. Behaving in an ethical manner also includes respecting the patient's rights, such as the right to privacy and confidentiality. Ethical behavior also includes remembering that not everyone behaves with the same values and ideals and respecting them for their differences.

Ethical decision making

Steps in the ethical decision making process
1. Identify the health problem.
2. Define the ethical issue.
3. Gather additional information.
4. Delineate the decision maker.
5. Examine ethical and moral principles.
6. Explore alternative options.
7. Implement decisions.
8. Evaluate and modify actions.

Multicultural patients' needs

Respect and tolerate multicultural beliefs and values, even if your patient is non-verbal. Most patients and their families willingly share their beliefs, so do not be embarrassed to ask about their preferences. Ask your supervisor for multicultural sensitivity training. Obtain a guide from The Association of Multicultural Counseling and Development. Keep a list of translators' phone numbers. Speak slowly while facing the patient; do not address the translator first. Order translations of patient guides and forms. Post pictorial direction signs. Allow multicultural families as much latitude as possible, without causing undue stress for your other patients. If you anticipate that a ritual will be noisy or alarming for other patients, respectfully guide the family to the Quiet Room. Realize some cultures have beliefs about specific food having healing or soothing qualities. Stay alert for poisoning from traditional Chinese, Indian, Pacific Islander, and Mexican herbal medicines, which often contain mercury.

Important terms

- **Advance directive** - A legal document in which the patient communicates to his/her family and physician what kind of medical intervention he/she desires. A living will is a type of advance directive that terminally ill patients often make. Specific laws regarding advance directives vary by state, but the patient must always be competent.
- **Anatomical gift** - The Uniform Anatomical Gift Act of 1968 facilitates organ transplantation under one standard, which is important when organs are transported across state lines. The Act was revised in 1987 and 2006 to cover transplants from cadavers and fetuses only through the national Organ Procurement and Transplantation Network (OPTN). Organ donations from living donors have many ethical and legal pitfalls, and are addressed in separate laws by each state.
- **Arbitration agreement** - The patient agrees to give up the right to sue the doctor. An arbiter (arbitrator) awards damages if injury results. Settlement is faster for the patient, and the doctor gets a malpractice insurance discount. Both parties save on legal fees.
- **Assault** - The touching of another person with an intent to harm, without that person's consent, A willful attempt to illegally inflict injury on or threaten a person
- **Assault and battery** - Assault is declaring or threatening your intent to touch a patient inappropriately or to cause physical harm. Battery is the actual act of inappropriate touching.
- **Assumption of risk** - (A.) A defense against an accusation of negligence. The defendant states the situation was obviously hazardous, so the complainant should have realized injury could result. (B.) An insurance company takes the risk of extending coverage, realizing the policyholder might make a claim, but it is statistically more likely to make a profit from the premiums.
- **Breach of confidentiality** - Occurs when information that should be kept secret, with access limited to appropriate persons, is given to an inappropriate person
- **Code blue** - The adult patient is in cardiac arrest. Call the resuscitation team immediately. Sometimes called Code 10. Code Pink refers to infant cardiac arrest.
- **Comparative negligence** - A rule used in accident cases to calculate the percentage of responsibility of each person (joint tortfeasors) directly involved in the accident. Damages (money compensation) are awarded based on a complex formula.
- **Consent to release information** - Patient's signature authorizes release of health information between provider and other entities, such as third party payers. Design of this form should be carefully considered, and may include language translation (verbal and/or written).
- **Consent to treatment** - Required for all treatment, unless the patient is unconscious or an unaccompanied minor in an emergency. Patient agrees to receive basic, routine services, diagnostic procedures, and medical care.
- **Contributory negligence** - If a person is injured partially because of his/her own negligence — even if it is slight — then the person who caused the accident does not pay any damages (money) to the injured person. Forty-four states recognize that applying the rule of contributory negligence could lead to unfair acquittal of genuinely negligent defendants, so they now use a comparative negligence test as a more balanced approach. In the 6 states that still have contributory negligence rules, juries tend to ignore it as unfair.

- Defamation - Defaming a person exposes him or her to public ridicule or tarnishes his or her memory through untrue and malicious statements. The defamed person can lose business due to loss of his or her good name.
- DNR order - "Do Not Resuscitate", a type of advance directive. A DNR order must be written in the patient's chart by the attending physician in order to be valid. All discussions with the patient and the family should be clearly documented in the chart. In the absence of a written DNR order, call a full Code Blue and proceed with resuscitation.
- Fraud - An intentional perversion of truth; deceitful practice or device resorted to with intent to deprive another of property or other right; intentional dishonesty for unfair or illegal gain.
- Invasion of privacy - Unsolicited or unauthorized exposure of patient information.
- Libel - A written statement that harms an individual's character, name, or reputation. A defamatory libel statement may be true, but is published maliciously (without just cause).
- Malpractice - Professional misconduct, resulting in failure to provide due care. Most malpractice lawsuits are related to professional negligence, the failure to perform what is considered standard care.
- MPI - Master patient index, a database associating the patient's name with his/her unique identifier. A unique identifier is assigned for confidentiality, security and filing accuracy. A unique identifier can be a medical record number (MRN), specimen, number, study number, or insurance number.
- Negligence - Taking an unreasonable, careless action that could foreseeably cause harm. Failing to exercise due care for others that a prudent, reasonable person would do. Negligence is accidental. Negligence is not an intentional tort, such as trespass or assault. Business errors, miscalculations, and failure to act can be negligent.
- Registration record - Sufficient demographic information is collected before service is rendered, including name, address, date of birth, next of kin, payment arrangements, and a unique patient identification number.
- Reportable incident - A dangerous event that must be reported to the supervisor or Safety Officer within a specific time frame, usually 24 hours to 5 days. Reportable incidents include:
  - Medication errors
  - Failure to assess and treat a patient according to state protocols, especially if it results in serious injury or death
  - Injuries or death while in care (e.g., attempted suicide)
  - Inappropriate use of a device or drug that results in death or injury
  - Motor vehicle accident resulting in death or injury
  - Suspicion of drug or alcohol abuse by a healthcare provider
  - Acts or omissions that threaten public safety or result in poor patient outcome
- Slander - Oral statements that damage someone's reputation. It is a form of defamation.
- Statute of limitations - A law defining the maximum period the complainant or appellant can wait before filing a lawsuit. The limitation date varies according to the type of case and if it falls within state or federal jurisdiction. Usually, the limitation is 1 to 6 years. Homicide has no limitation. If the complainant misses the deadline, then the right to sue is "stats barred" (dead). Rarely, a judge will "toll" (extend) the

deadline if the injury was discovered late or a trusted person hid misuse of funds or failure to pay. Minors' rights to bring negligence charges are tolled until the age of 18.

- Subpoena duces tecum - Subpoena duces tecum literally means bring [it] with you under penalty of punishment. It is a court order for a witness to produce documents. The judge must carefully consider if subpoena duces tecum transgresses the patient's HIPAA rights.
- Tort - An injury or wrong committed, either with or without force, to the person or property of another, for which civil liability may be imposed.
- Vicarious liability - When a person is held responsible for the tort of another even though the person being held responsible may not have done anything wrong. This is often the case with employers who are held vicariously liable for the damages caused by their employees.

ECG

Layers of the heart

Three layers of tissue form the heart wall. The outer layer of the heart wall is the epicardium, the middle layer is the myocardium, and the inner layer is the endocardium:
- Epicardium- the membrane that covers the outside of the heart
- Myocardium-The muscular wall of the heart, the thickest of the three layers of the heart wall, it lies between the inner layer (endocardium) and the outer layer (epicardium).
- Endocardium- membrane lining the inside surface of heart

Heart chambers and valves

Heart chambers

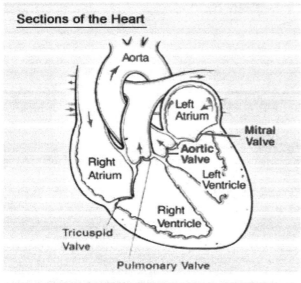

Electrical conduction system

Electrical impulses from your heart muscle (the myocardium) cause your heart to beat (contract). This electrical signal begins in the sinoatrial (SA) node, located at the top of the right atrium. The SA node is sometimes called the heart's "natural pacemaker." When an electrical impulse is released from this natural pacemaker, it causes the atria to contract. The signal then passes through the atrioventricular (AV) node. The AV node checks the signal and sends it through the muscle fibers of the ventricles, causing them to contract. The SA node sends electrical impulses at a certain rate, but your heart rate may still change depending on physical demands, stress or hormonal factors.

Relationship to ECG
The electrical conduction system of the heart generates and propagates the electrical impulses that sustain the rhythmic electrical contractions of the heart. The entire system is

composed of the sinoatrial (SA) and atrioventricular (AV) nodes and the internodal pathways, the Bundle of His, as well as the right and left bundle branches and the anterior and posterior fascicles. First, the SA node generates a spontaneous electrical impulse that stimulates atrial contraction, corresponding to the P wave on the ECG. Next, the electrical impulse reaches the AV node and slows in velocity. This corresponds to the PR segment on the ECG. The electrical impulse travels through the Bundle of His and the bundle braches, then to the Purkinje fibers. The Purkinje fibers carry the electrical impulse that stimulate the ventricles to depolarize and contract, corresponding to the QRS complex.

Cardiac cycle

Ventricular Systole:
1. ventricles contract
2. ventricular contraction regulated by AV node
3. semilunar valves (to aorta & pulmonary arteries) open
4. atrioventricular valves close ("lub")

Ventricular Diastole:
1. ventricles relax, atria contract
2. atrial contraction regulated by SA node (pacemaker)
3. semilunar valves close ("dupp")
4. atrioventricular valves open

ECG tracing of a cardiac cycle
P wave represents the Atrial depolarization
QRS complex represents the Ventricular depolarization
T wave represents the ventricular repolarization

Heart sounds

A heartbeat is a two-part pumping action that takes about a second. As blood collects in the upper chambers (the right and left atria), the heart's natural pacemaker (the SA node) sends out an electrical signal that causes the atria to contract. This contraction pushes blood through the tricuspid and mitral valves into the resting lower chambers (the right and left ventricles). This part of the two-part pumping phase (the longer of the two) is called the diastole. The second part of the pumping phase begins when the ventricles are full of blood. The electrical signals from the SA node travel along a pathway of cells to the ventricles, causing them to contract. This is called systole. As the tricuspid and mitral valves shut tight to prevent a back flow of blood; the pulmonary and aortic valves are pushed open. While blood is pushed from the right ventricle into the lungs to pick up oxygen, oxygen-rich blood flows from the left ventricle to the heart and other parts of the body. After blood moves into the pulmonary artery and the aorta, the ventricles relax, and the pulmonary and aortic valves close. The lower pressure in the ventricles causes the tricuspid and mitral valves to open, and the cycle begins again. This series of contractions is repeated over and over again, increasing during times of exertion and decreasing while at rest.

ECG

An electrocardiograph machine records the heart's electrical activity on an electrocardiogram (ECG or ECG). The ECG monitors heart rate, patterns of heartbeats, the

- 35 -

size and location of the chambers of the heart, and helps to diagnose heart conditions. The ECG is a non-invasive, painless, inexpensive way to determine if there is any damage to the heart muscle (myocardium) or electrical conduction system. The cardiologist uses the ECG to determine if drug therapy or pacemaker implants are having the desired effect. The P wave on an ECG corresponds to the atria contracting. The QRS complex corresponds to the ventricles contracting. The T wave is repolarization. For a resting ECG, position the patient lying down, face up. If the patient has difficulty breathing (dyspnea), prop the patient's head up with pillows. For a stress test, 12—15 leads are attached to the patient, who runs on a treadmill. For a Holter monitor, 3—5 leads are used, and the results of the ECG are recorded on a telemetry device worn around the patient's neck for 24—48 hours.

ECG leads

During an ECG, electrodes, or leads, are placed at various locations on the body and record electrical activity of the heart. Typically, 12 leads are used: three standard leads, three augmented leads, and six precordial leads. The standard and augmented leads view the heart from a frontal plane and the precordial leads view the heart from a horizontal plane. The standard leads are bipolar and contain one positive and one negative electrode. Augmented leads are unipolar and contain one positive electrode. Precordial leads are also unipolar with only one electrode.

An ECG lead is the wire and electrode that connects the patient to the electrocardiograph machine (also abbreviated ECG). A standard 12-lead ECG actually has only 10 wires and electrodes, which record 12 electrical vectors:
Unipolar Leads:
- Augmented Vector Right (AVR) [right atrial view]
- Augmented Vector Left (AVL) [lateral view]
- Augmented Vector Foot (AVF) [inferior view]
- Precordial chest lead V1 [anterior view]
- Precordial chest lead V2 [anterior view]
- Precordial chest lead V3 [septal view]
- Precordial chest lead V4 [septal view]
- Precordial chest lead V5 [lateral view]
- Precordial chest lead V6 [lateral view]

Bipolar Leads:
- Limb lead I [lateral view]
- Limb lead II [inferior view]
- Limb lead III [inferior view]

Rarely, a cardiologist who suspects damage to the rear wall of the heart that is not evident on a 12-lead will ask for V8 and V9 on the patient's back.

Bipolar ECG leads
The three standard leads used in ECG measurement are bipolar leads. They contain one positive and one negative electrode. The ECG measures the difference in electrical potential recorded by each electrode. Lead I is placed on the right arm (negative electrode) and left arm (positive electrode.) Lead II is placed on the right arm (negative) and left leg (positive.) Lead III is placed on the left arm (negative) and left leg (positive.)

Einthoven's Law describes their placement and mathematical relationship to one another. The standard leads view the heart's activity in a frontal place.

Unipolar ECG leads
The three augmented ECG leads are unipolar leads. They contain only one positive electrode and are placed at the right arm, left arm, and left leg. They are termed aVR (augmented voltage of the right arm), aVL (augmented voltage of the left arm), and aVF (augmented voltage of the left foot). The electrodes record the electrical potential at one point in reference to the other two leads. For example, the right arm is positive in reference to the left arm and left leg. This electrode records electrical activity in the heart from the right-sided direction. The augmented leads view the heart's activity in a frontal place.

Precordial ECG leads
Six precordial leads are used in ECG measurement. The leads are unipolar and have only one positive electrode. The leads are placed across the chest horizontally. This allows the heart's activity to be viewed in a horizontal plane rather than a frontal plane, as with the standard and augmented leads. Leads V1 and V2 are placed over the right ventricle, at the 4th intercostal space, on the right and left sides of the sternum, respectively. Lead V4 is placed at the 5th intercostal space on the midclavicular line. Lead V3 lies in between V2 and V4. Leads V5 and V6 are placed over the left ventricle at the 5th intercostal space, at the anterior axillary line and the midaxillary line, respectively.

Einthoven's triangle and law

The three standard, bipolar, leads form a triangle over the body. They are placed at the right arm, left arm, and left leg. The three leads exhibit a mathematical relationship to one another. As described by Einthoven, the electrical potential (height and depth) of ECG measurements on Lead I plus those on Lead III equal the electrical potential of the measurements on Lead II. Given this law, if the values of the electrical potential at any two points of the triangle are known, the third value can be calculated

Placement of ECG leads in dextrocardia

Dextrocardia is a condition in which the heart is located on the right side of the chest instead of the left. Further, the heart's chambers are reversed, with the right chambers appearing on the left side of the heart and the left chambers appearing on the right side of the heart. Often this is associated with situs inversus, a condition in which all body organs are in mirror image placement to the normal orientation. In this situation, all leads for an ECG must be placed in the mirror image of traditional electrode positioning. The right arm and right leg electrodes should be placed on the left arm and leg, respectively. Also, the chest leads should be placed in the same orientation as a normal ECG, but on the right side of the chest rather than the left.

ECG calibration

It is important to always check that the ECG equipment is calibrated before recording an ECG tracing. If the machine is not properly calibrated, the results of the tracing cannot be considered accurate. First, the speed of the paper should be 25 millimeters per second. Therefore, each one-millimeter square is equal to 0.04 seconds (40 milliseconds.) Also, ten one-millimeter squares measured vertically, equal one milliVolt of electrical charge. If the one milliVolt calibration button is pressed on an ECG machine, a square-shaped signal should appear over approximately 10 millimeters horizontally and 10 millimeters vertically. If this does not appear on the ECG tracing, the machine is incorrectly calibrated.

Standard paper speed
Normal ECG paper speed is 25 millimeters per second. Time on an ECG is measured horizontally, with each small, one-millimeter square of the graph paper corresponding to 0.04 seconds or 40 milliseconds. Each large square, composed of five one-millimeter squares and marked with thicker grid lines, corresponds to 0.20 seconds or 200 milliseconds. Therefore, five large squares equal one second in duration. The accurate measurement of time on an ECG is important in determining heart rate and the length of various intervals in the cardiac cycle.

Troubleshooting in ECG interpretation

Errors in the recording of the ECG tracing may lead to incorrect or incomplete diagnosis of cardiovascular disease. This may lead to unnecessary, insufficient, or improper treatment of the patient. When interpreting and ECG tracing, it is important to analyze all factors that may have led to a recording error. First, recognize potential sources of artifact or interference. These sources may vary, depending on the type of ECG performed and the location. Second, verify that all equipment is in proper, working condition. Third, analyze the placement of leads on the patient and confirm that skin characteristics did not cause the loss of electrode contact. Factors affecting the quality of an ECG tracing should be analyzed in order to report accurate ECG results.

Single- and multi-channel ECG printouts

ECG machines are available with a variety of features, including multiple options for ECG printers. Most ECG machines are able to interpret the information from the 12 limb leads and print in three, four, six, or twelve channel printouts. Single-channel printouts are simpler, producing only one tracing. Single channel printouts are less sophisticated and used for less advanced diagnostic application. More than one channel is usually needed to fully interpret the heart's function.

NSR, SA, AV, pacemaker, block , and arrhythmia

A normal sinus rhythm (NSR) on an ECG denotes that the electrical impulses start in the sinoatrial node (SA) first, and cause the right and left atria to contract simultaneously to effectively pump blood into the ventricles. The contraction of the atria is followed by contraction of the ventricles, which move blood throughout the body. The conduction system coordinates the contractions. If the SA node does not initiate the electrical impulse, the atrioventricular node (AV) can do so. However, the AV node is not as capable of increasing the heart rate as is the SA node, because the AV resting rate is lower than that of the SA node. The patient requires a mechanical pacemaker to fix the slow heart rate. All of the cells of the heart are capable of generating the electrical impulses necessary to trigger a heartbeat; this property is known as automaticity. Signal conduction problems, termed block, can occur at any site along the conduction pathway, causing an arrhythmia, which is an alteration in the normal rhythm.

ECG recording errors

Errors in the recording of the ECG tracing may lead to incorrect or incomplete diagnosis of cardiovascular disease. This may lead to unnecessary, insufficient, or improper treatment of the patient. When interpreting and ECG tracing, it is important to analyze all factors that may have led to a recording error. These factors may be incorrect calibration or standardization of the ECG equipment, incorrect paper speed, lead reversals, or incorrect lead placement. Troubleshooting techniques before and after the recording of the ECG should be employed to ensure accurate reporting of ECG results.

Right and left arm lead reversal
Interchanging the right and left arm leads is an easily recognizable error in ECG recording. Care should be taken to note that when the patient is on the ECG exam table, his right arm is on the left side of the table, and vice versa. If these leads are reversed, lead I will show an inverted P wave and a negative QRS complex. The T wave may or may not be affected. Also, if the QRS complex appears inverted in lead I compared to V6, the arm leads are most likely reversed. In addition, lead II will have the appearance of a normal lead III and lead III will have the appearance of lead II. Similarly the appearance of aVR will mimic a normal aVL recording, and the aVL will mimic aVR.

Right arm and right leg lead reversal
Interchanging the right arm and right leg electrodes is recognized on an ECG as an isoelectric lead II. In properly placed electrodes, lead II detects a voltage difference between the electrical potential of the left leg and the right arm. If the right arm and leg electrodes are reversed, then lead II will detect a voltage difference between the right leg and the left leg. The potential in the legs is virtually the same, so lead II will show a recording with almost no activity. Based on Einthoven's Law, the sum of the potential in leads I and III is equal to that in lead II. Therefore, if lead II is essentially zero in reversed right arm and right leg electrodes, leads I and III will produce mirror-image tracings of each other.

Left arm and left leg lead reversal
Interchanging the left arm and left leg electrodes is a difficult error to detect on an ECG tracing. In this case, lead III will produce an inverted tracing compared to normal tracings. Also, lead aVL will be interpreted as aVF and aVF will be interpreted as aVL. Similarly, lead I will be interpreted as lead II and lead II will be interpreted as lead I. Often, this problem is not discovered until multiple ECG recordings from the same patient have been analyzed and the differences in tracings can be noted.

Left arm and right leg lead reversal
If the left arm and right leg electrodes are interchanged, lead III will be virtually isoelectric, exhibiting almost no electrical activity. Based on Einthoven's Law, the sum of the electrical potential in leads I and III equals the potential in lead II. If the potential in lead III is zero, then leads I and II will have nearly identical appearances on the ECG tracing. Similarly, leads aVF and aVL will resemble each other.

Right arm and left leg lead reversal
Interchanging the right arm and left leg electrodes is an extremely uncommon error in ECG recording. However, in this instance, lead aVF will resemble a normal aVR and lead aVR will resemble aVF. The P wave, then, in aVF will be abnormally inverted. These atypical findings on the ECG tracing can lead to an incorrect diagnosis of myocardial infarction.

Incorrect placement of chest leads V1 and V2

Proper placement of lead V1 and V2 requires accurate identification of the fourth intercostal space. If these leads are not accurately positioned, recording anomalies will be noted in all precordial leads. Most likely, leads V1 and V2 will be positioned too high, near the third intercostal space. These leads will then exhibit inverted P and T waves. The leads will also exhibit an R wave after the S wave. These same anomalies are found in right ventricular enlargement, with the exception of the inverted P wave. Care should be taken to distinguish diagnostic abnormalities from recording errors. Also, if leads V1 and V2 are placed incorrectly, the ECG tracing will appear to exhibit signs of right bundle branch block – a widened QRS interval and an ST segment that sloped into the T wave.

Incorrect placement of chest leads V2 and V3

Reversing the placement of precordial leads V2 and V3 will produce abnormal R waves on an ECG. In a normal ECG tracing, the amplitude of the R wave increases from leads V2 to V3 to V4. If this progression is not seen, the leads are most likely misplaced. Also in this case, the S wave in lead V3 will appear larger than the S wave in lead V2.

Incorrect paper speed

The standard ECG tracing is set to a paper speed of 25 millimeters per second. This speed allows for accurate measurement of all crucial and diagnostic waveforms without distorting low amplitude waves. If the paper speed is not set to 25 millimeters per second, the actual speed should be noted on the tracing. If the paper speed is incorrectly set and the speed is not noted, errors will occur in the determination of heart rate, heart rhythm, and size of waveforms.

Electrical interference in recording ECGs

In ECG recording, the quality of the tracing can be influenced by outside interference, or influences that do not originate from the heart muscle. These influences or interferences are called artifacts and are commonly caused by electrical interference, somatic muscle tremor, and a wandering baseline. The presence of any artifact makes accurate measurement and interpretation of the cardiac cycle difficult. Electrical interference as an artifact may originate from internal or external sources. In the case of external electrical interference, the interference arises from an electrical current near the patient, usually 50 to 60 Hertz in frequency. Straightening the leads so the wires are aligned with the patient's body can minimize this artifact.

Somatic tremor in recording ECGs

In ECG recording, the quality of the tracing can be influenced by outside interference, or influences that do not originate from the heart muscle. These influences or interferences are called artifacts and are commonly caused by electrical interference, somatic muscle tremor, and a wandering baseline. The presence of any artifact makes accurate measurement and interpretation of the cardiac cycle difficult. A somatic muscle tremor is known as an internal electrical interference. This artifact originates within the patient's body as a tremor, shiver, hiccup, or other tense or moving muscles. The ECG tracing will display a "noisy baseline" is the presence of tense or a somatic tremor.

Artifacts in ECG recording

In ECG recording, the quality of the tracing can be influenced by outside interference, or influences that do not originate from the heart muscle. These influences or interferences are called artifacts. These interferences may be caused by factors within the body of the patient or by external factors. Common physiologic factors, arising from the patient himself, include any muscle movements or spasms, electrodes placed over a pulsating vessel, sweat on the skin, and respiratory interference. Common external causes include the loose connection of an electrode, the presence of an alternating current from equipment or power lines near the patient, and movements in the environment during the ECG recording. The presence of any artifact makes accurate measurement and interpretation of the cardiac cycle difficult.

Wandering or shifting baseline

The presence of any artifact makes accurate measurement and interpretation of the cardiac cycle difficult. A wandering or shifting baseline on an ECG tracing is the result of poor electrode contact on the patient's skin. To ensure proper electrode contact, the patient's skin must be clean, dry, and contain no abnormalities or abrasions at the lead site. Also, sites with excessive body hair or oily skin may interfere with good electrode contact. A wandering baseline occurs gradually over the length of the ECG tracing, while a shifting baseline occurs abruptly with sudden loss of contact between the electrode and the patient's skin.

Electrical hazards

Most hazards and accidents from electrical equipment come from fire and electrical shock. These hazards are present due to the use of damaged equipment or damaged cords or wall sockets. A cord should always be inspected before plugging it in to a socket. If the cord or socket is cracked, exposed, or otherwise damaged, leakage of electrical current could occur and harm persons near the cord or socket. Always have equipment turned off when plugging it in to a socket. Further, never pull the cord to unplug equipment; pull the plug from the wall socket. Do not place cords near hot or sharp objects.

Leakage current

Leakage current is the electrical current that flows through the ground conductor. It is present in all operating electrical equipment, often in very small amounts. If a ground conductor is not present, the leakage current could flow to any conductive surface, including the human body. For medical equipment, the requirements for maximum current leakage are maintained necessarily low to prevent patient hazards. Electrical cords and wires are also insulated to ensure protection against current leakage.

Electrical shock

Electric shock is a common hazard associated with the use of damaged electrical equipment. An electric shock may cause minor burns or skin irritation, burns to internal organs, or cause the heart to stop beating. Further, symptoms of electric shock include difficulties breathing, an irregular heartbeat, or unconsciousness. Electric shock can cause sudden death.

Ground connectors to prevent electrical hazards

Ground connectors divert extraneous or leakage electrical current to the ground or earth. Ground connectors are made of conductive material to draw the current away from other materials that may prove hazardous, like the human body. Leakage current is present in all operating electrical equipment, but it is safely managed and electrical shock is prevented by the use of protective grounding techniques.

Extinguishing an electrical fire

Fire is a common hazard associated with the use of damaged electrical equipment. If electrical equipment, cords, or sockets begin smoking, sparking, or catch fire, turn off the device and unplug it. Call 911 if a fire ignites. A fire extinguisher appropriate for electrical fires should be kept in any space in which electrical equipment is being used. Class "C" fire extinguishers are appropriate for electrical fires. Baking soda may be used to extinguish small electrical fires. Water should never be used to extinguish electrical fires. Water is a conductor of electricity and could lead to electric shocks.

Important terms

- Cardiac output - The volume of blood being pumped by the heart in a minute. It is equal to the heart rate multiplied by the stroke volume.
- Heart rate - The number of contractions of the heart in one minute. It is measured in beats per minute (bpm). When resting, the adult human heart beats at about 70 bpm (males) and 75 bpm (females), but this rate varies between people.
- Stroke volume - The amount of blood ejected by the ventricle of the heart with each beat, usually expressed in milliliters (ml).

Basic Anatomy and Physiology

Abdominal quadrants and body planes

The four abdominal quadrants are:
- Right Upper Quadrant (RUQ)
- Left Upper Quadrant (LUQ)
- Right Lower Quadrant (RLQ)
- Left Lower Quadrant (LLQ)

The transverse plane divides the patient's body into imaginary upper (superior) and lower (inferior or caudal) halves. The sagittal plane divides the body, or any body part, vertically into right and left sections. The sagittal plane runs parallel to the midline of the body. Equal halves are the midsagittal plane. The median plane divides the body into right and left halves. The median plane runs vertically through the midline of the body, or any body structure. The median plane is a type of sagittal plane. The coronal plane divides the body, or any body structure, into front and back (anterior and posterior sections). The coronal plane runs vertically through the body at right angles to the midline. The coronal plane is also called anterior or frontal plane. The posterior plane is the back, also called dorsal or ventral.

Body systems

The 11 body systems and their functions are as follows:
- Cardiovascular - Pumps blood throughout the body via the heart and blood vessels
- Digestive - Transforms food to energy and eliminates solid waste
- Endocrine - Releases hormones into the bloodstream to control metabolism, growth, and reproduction
- Excretory - Also called urinary; removes waste products from the blood and expels it from the body
- Immune - Defends against all foreign substances
- Integumentary - Skin prevents moisture loss, regulates temperature, protects from sunburn, and senses pain, pressure, touch, hot and cold
- Muscular - Skeletal muscles move the body; smooth muscle works internal organs; cardiac muscle pumps blood
- Nervous - Controls movement, memory, senses, and communicates with the outside world
- Reproductive - Allows continuation of the human species and differentiates the sexes
- Respiratory - Gas exchange (oxygen intake and carbon dioxide expulsion)
- Skeletal - Supports and shapes; protects internal organs; stores minerals; produces blood cells

Digestive system

The main parts of the digestive system in order of how food passes through them are listed and explained below:

1. Digestion starts in the mouth with the action of saliva containing amylase to start starch digestion. The mouth also contains the hard and the soft palates.
2. The 20 primary or 32 permanent teeth are used for mastication of food
3. The tongue holds the taste buds and moves the food towards the esophagus.
4. The pharynx connects the mouth to the esophagus. The epiglottis keeps food from entering the trachea. The pharynx is about 5 inches long.
5. The esophagus is a 12" tube leading to the stomach. Peristaltic waves start here and moves food into the stomach.
6. The stomach sac is controlled by the lower esophageal sphincter at the top and the pyloric sphincter at the bottom. Food mixes with hydrochloric acid in the stomach to make chyme. Food normally stays in the stomach for 2-4 hours.
7. The small intestine contains the duodenum (10"), jejunum (8'), and ileum (12'). The majority of digestion takes place in the duodenum. The small intestine receives bile, produced by the liver and stored in the gall bladder, to digest fats, and amylase and insulin from the pancreas to break down starches and sugars. Digestion in the small intestine can take between 3 and 10 hours.
8. The large intestine absorbs water and salts. The large intestine consists of the cecum (with vermiform appendix); ascending, transverse, descending, and sigmoid colon, the rectum and anus for defecation. The ileocecal valve prevents food from reentering the small intestine.

Total digestion can take between 24 hours and 3 days.

Skeletal system

There are about 206 bones in the human body, they function to protect and preserve the shape of soft tissues. The skeleton provides a framework for the muscles, it controls and directs internal pressure and provides stability anchoring points for other soft tissues. There are a wide variety of bones/bony tissues adapted for specific functions to aid locomotion and support; bones are moved by the skeletal muscles. In addition the skeletal system stores and produces blood cells in the bone marrow.

Skeletal system structures
There are two types of bone tissue: compact and spongy. The names imply that the two types differ in density, or how tightly the tissue is packed together. There are three types of cells that contribute to bone homeostasis. Osteoblasts are bone-forming cell, osteoclasts resorb or break down bone, and osteocytes are mature bone cells. Equilibrium between osteoblasts and osteoclasts maintains bone tissue.

Compact bone
Compact bone consists of closely packed osteons or haversian systems. The osteon consists of a central canal called the osteonic (haversian) canal, which is surrounded by concentric rings (lamellae) of matrix. Between the rings of matrix, the bone cells (osteocytes) are located in spaces called lacunae. Small channels (canaliculi) radiate from the lacunae to the osteonic (haversian) canal to provide passageways through the hard matrix. In compact

bone, the haversian systems are packed tightly together to form what appears to be a solid mass. The osteonic canals contain blood vessels that are parallel to the long axis of the bone. These blood vessels interconnect, by way of perforating canals, with vessels on the surface of the bone.

<u>Spongy bone</u>
Spongy (cancellous) bone is lighter and less dense than compact bone. Spongy bone consists of plates (trabeculae) and bars of bone adjacent to small, irregular cavities that contain red bone marrow. The canaliculi connect to the adjacent cavities, instead of a central haversian canal, to receive their blood supply. It may appear that the trabeculae are arranged in a haphazard manner, but they are organized to provide maximum strength similar to braces that are used to support a building. The trabeculae of spongy bone follow the lines of stress and can realign if the direction of stress changes.

<u>Bones and joints</u>
- Head: Cranium made of 8 bones including the frontal (forehead), 2 parietal (back), occipital (back), 2 temporal (side), sphenoid (base of skull), and ethmoid (nasal cavity). There are14 facial bones: mandibular (lower jaw), 2 maxilla (upper jaw), 2 lacrimal (inner side of orbital cavity), 2 nasal conchae, 2 turbinate, vomer), and 2 zygoma (cheek) bones, and 2 palate bones. The ear has 6 bones including malleus (hammer), incus (anvil) and stapes (stirrup) bones in each ear
- Spine: 7 cervical (neck), 12 thoracic (upper back), and 5 lumbar (lower back) vertebrae, the sacrum (rump), and coccyx (tail bone)
- Chest: Ribs, sternum, scapula (shoulder blade), and clavicle (collar bone)
- Pelvis: Ilium (upper), ischium (lower), pubis (front), and 2 coxal (hip)
- Arms: Humerus (upper), radius and ulna (forearm), carpals (wrist), metacarpals (hand), phalanges (fingers)
- Legs: Femur (thigh), patella (knee), tibia and fibula (calf), tarsals (ankle), metatarsals (front foot), calcaneous (heel), phalanges (toes)
- Diarthrotic articulations: Moveable joints with synovial fluid, cartilage cushions, held together by ligaments, like the limbs
- Synarthrotic articulations: Immovable joints like the spine and skull

<u>Cartilage, ligament, and tendon</u>
Cartilage is a dense connective tissue composed of collagen and/or elastin fibers on the end of bones, which provides a smooth surface for articulation by reducing friction. Hyaline cartilage contains chondrocytes that make it look glassy, and is found in the nose, larynx, trachea, ribs and sternum. Hyaline cartilage makes an embryo's skeleton. Elastic cartilage contains elastin, which makes it yellow, and is found in the outer ear (pinna) and epiglottis. Fibrocartilage is composed of strands of fibers that function to help limit movement and prevent bones from rubbing together. Fibrocartilage is found in the knee, the pubic bones in the pelvic region and between the vertebrae in the spine.

A ligament is a fibrous band composed of connective tissue stretching from one bone to another in a joint to provide lateral stability. Ligaments also connect cartilages and other structures. Injuries to ligaments are sprains, which are slow to heal and may require physiotherapy and surgery.

A tendon is also called a sinew, and connects muscle to bone. Tendons grow into the bone and make mineralized connections with the bone. Tendons transform muscle contraction into joint movement. Tendons can withstand great pressure, but tendons that tear do not heal well. A complete tear requires surgical repair. Damage to a tendon and its muscle in a joint is a strain. Tendonitis is inflammation of the tendon.

Muscular system

The muscular system is composed of specialized cells called muscle fibers. Muscle fibers' predominant function is contractibility. Muscles, where attached to bones or internal organs and blood vessels, are responsible for movement. Nearly all movement in the body is the result of muscle contraction. The muscular system in humans consists of three different types of muscles: cardiac, skeletal and smooth. Cardiac muscle is a striated muscle that makes up the heart. It is the only type of muscle consisting of branching fibers. Skeletal muscle consists of voluntary muscles attached to the frame of the skeletal system enabling bodily movement. Smooth muscle is the involuntary muscle that enables the movement of internal organs. Movement of most muscles is controlled through the nervous system, although some muscles (such as cardiac muscle) can be completely autonomous. There are about 70,000 muscles in the human body

Skeletal muscle
The functional characteristics of a skeletal muscle cell:
- The cell membrane is called the sarcolemma. This membrane is structured to receive and conduct stimuli. The sarcoplasm of the cell is filled with contractile myofibrils and this results in the nuclei and other organelles being relegated to the edge of the cell.
- Myofibrils are contractile units within the cell which consist of a regular array of protein myofilaments. Each myofilament runs longitudinally with respect to the muscle fiber. There are two types: the thick bands and the thin bands. Thick bands are made of multiple molecules of a protein called myosin.
- The thin bands are made of multiple molecules of a protein called actin. The thin actin bands are attached to a Z-line or Z-disk of an elastic protein called titin. The titin protein also extends into the myofibril anchoring the other bands in position. From each Z-line to the next is a unit called the sarcomere.

Reproductive system

The major function of the reproductive system is to ensure survival of the species. This is carried out by the four following objectives:
- To produce egg and sperm cells
- To transport and sustain these cells
- To nurture the developing offspring
- To produce hormones

Digestive system

The digestive system includes the digestive tract and its accessory organs, which process food into molecules that can be absorbed and utilized by the cells of the body. Food is broken down, bit by bit, until the molecules are small enough to be absorbed and the waste products are eliminated. The digestive tract, also called the alimentary canal or gastrointestinal (GI) tract, consists of a long continuous tube that extends from the mouth to the anus. It includes the mouth, pharynx, esophagus, stomach, small intestine, and large intestine. The tongue and teeth are accessory structures located in the mouth. The Salivary glands, liver, and gallbladder pancreas are major accessory organs that have a role in digestion. These organs secrete fluids into the digestive tract.

The six main functions of the digestive system are as follows:
- Ingestion - The first activity of the digestive system is to take in food through the mouth. This process, called ingestion, has to take place before anything else can happen.
- Mechanical digestion - The large pieces of food that are ingested have to be broken into smaller particles that can be acted upon by various enzymes. This is mechanical digestion, which begins in the mouth with chewing or mastication and continues with churning and mixing actions in the stomach.
- Chemical digestion - The complex molecules of carbohydrates, proteins, and fats are transformed by chemical digestion into smaller molecules that can be absorbed and utilized by the cells. Chemical digestion, through a process called hydrolysis, uses water and digestive enzymes to break down the complex molecules. Digestive enzymes speed up the hydrolysis process, which is otherwise very slow.
- Movements - After ingestion and mastication, the food particles move from the mouth into the pharynx, then into the esophagus. This movement is deglutition or swallowing. Mixing movements occur in the stomach as a result of smooth muscle contraction. These repetitive contractions usually occur in small segments of the digestive tract and mix the food particles with enzymes and other fluids. The movements that propel the food particles through the digestive tract are called peristalsis. These are rhythmic waves of contractions that move the food particles through the various regions in which mechanical and chemical digestion takes place.
- Absorption - The simple molecules that result from chemical digestion pass through cell membranes of the lining in the small intestine into the blood or lymph capillaries. This process is called absorption.
- Elimination - The food molecules that cannot be digested or absorbed need to be eliminated from the body. The removal of indigestible wastes through the anus, in the form of feces, is defecation or elimination.

Endocrine system

The endocrine system functions in the regulation of body activities. The endocrine system acts through chemical messengers called hormones that influence growth, development, and metabolic activities. The action of the endocrine system is measured in minutes, hours, or weeks. The endocrine system works with the nervous system to maintain homeostasis in the body. There are two major categories of glands in the body - exocrine and endocrine. Exocrine glands have ducts that carry their secretory product to a surface. These glands include the sweat, sebaceous, and mammary glands and, the glands that secrete digestive enzymes. The endocrine glands do not have ducts to carry their product to a surface. They are called ductless glands. The word endocrine is derived from the Greek terms "endo," meaning within, and "krine," meaning to separate or secrete. The secretory products of endocrine glands are called hormones and are secreted directly into the blood and then carried throughout the body where they influence only those cells that have receptor sites for that hormone.

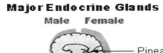

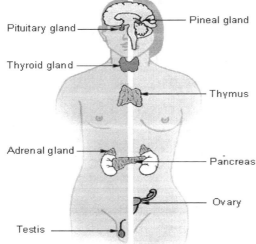

Hormones
Listed below are the major hormones and diseases that relate to each gland:

Gland	Hormones	Disease
Adrenal Cortex	Aldosterone Cortisol, androgens	Addison's Disease Cushing's Disease
Adrenal Medulla	Epinephrine Norepinephrine	Anxiety attacks Depression
Anterior Pituitary	Adrenocorticotropic hormone(ACTH) Follicle-stimulating hormone (FSH) Gonadotropic hormones Growth hormone (GH) Luteinizing hormone (LH) Prolactin Thyroid Stimulating Hormone (TSH)	Dwarfism Gigantism
Hypothalamus & Posterior Pituitary	Inhibiting hormones Antidiuretic hormone (ADH), Oxytocin Releasing hormones	Diabetes Insipidus
Kidneys	Calcitriol Erythropoietin	Hypertension
Ovaries	Estrogen Progesterone	Endometriosis Menometrorrhagia
Pancreas	Insulin Glucagon	Diabetes Mellitus
Parathyroid	Parathyroid hormone	Tetany Renal calculi

Gland	Hormones	Disease
Pineal	Melatonin	Alzheimer's Disease Jet lag
Testes	Testosterone	Gynecomastia Klinefelter Syndrome
Thymus	Thymic factor (TF) Thymosin Thymic humoral factor(THF) Thymopoietin	DiGeorge Syndrome
Thyroid	Calcitonin Thyroxine (T4) Triiodothyronine (T3)	Cretinism Goiter Myxedema
Digestive tract	Gastrin Cholecystokinin Secretin Ghrelin Motilin	Gastritis Gastroesophageal reflux

Growth hormone

Growth Hormone (GH, somatotropin) - controlled by both releasing and inhibiting hormones, GHRH and GHIH (somatostatin), from the hypothalamus. GH causes growth and development of the musculoskeletal system and other tissues. It stimulates amino acids to be used for protein synthesis and causes lipolysis to provide fatty acids for catabolism. For these reasons it is sometimes abused to stimulate muscle growth and catabolize fat. Negative feedback results from GH itself and also from mediators called somatomedins (Somatomedin is also known as Insulin-like Growth Factor 1) produced by the liver, muscles, and other tissue. Positive feedback is produced by strenuous exercise and energy demanding activities. Childhood hypersecretion of GH causes the excessive growth seen in gigantism, and adulthood hypersecretion causes acromegaly, a condition in which the bones are exaggerated in shape. Hyposecretion in childhood causes dwarfism.

Nervous system

The nervous system is the major controlling, regulatory, and communicating system in the body. It is the center of all mental activity including thought, learning, and memory. Together with the endocrine system, the nervous system is responsible for regulating and maintaining homeostasis. Through its receptors, the nervous system keeps us in touch with our environment, both external and internal. The three main functions of the nervous system are sensory, integrative and motor. Sensory part of the nervous system detects changes in the external environment like temperature, light and sound. It also monitors the internal environment such as blood pressure, pH, CO_2 level, and electrolyte levels. The input into the sensory system is called stimuli. Integration occurs when the stimuli from the sensory system is processed by the brain into create memories, thoughts, sensations, and decisions. Motor describes the response of the body due to the integration of the stimuli. This can result in the movement of a muscle or the release of a hormone from a gland.

Central nervous system

The brain and spinal cord are the organs of the central nervous system. Because they are so vitally important, the brain and spinal cord, located in the dorsal body cavity, are encased in bone for protection. The brain is in the cranial vault, and the spinal cord is in the vertebral canal of the vertebral column. Although considered to be two separate organs, the brain and spinal cord are continuous at the foramen magnum.

Peripheral nervous system

The organs of the peripheral nervous system are the nerves and ganglia. Nerves are bundles of nerve fibers, much like muscles are bundles of muscle fibers. Cranial nerves and spinal nerves extend from the CNS to peripheral organs such as muscles and glands. Ganglia are collections, or small knots, of nerve cell bodies outside the CNS. The peripheral nervous system is further subdivided into an afferent (sensory) division and an efferent (motor) division. The afferent or sensory division transmits impulses from peripheral organs to the CNS. The efferent or motor division transmits impulses from the CNS out to the peripheral organs to cause an effect or action. Finally, the efferent or motor division is again subdivided into the somatic nervous system and the autonomic nervous system. The somatic nervous system, also called the somatomotor or somatic efferent nervous system, supplies motor impulses to the skeletal muscles. Because these nerves permit conscious control of the skeletal muscles, it is sometimes called the voluntary nervous system. The autonomic nervous system, also called the visceral efferent nervous system, supplies motor impulses to cardiac muscle, to smooth muscle, and to glandular epithelium. It is further subdivided into sympathetic and parasympathetic divisions. Because the autonomic nervous system regulates involuntary or automatic functions, it is called the involuntary nervous system.

Neurons

Neurons are nerve cells that transmit nerve impulses throughout the central and peripheral nervous systems. The basic structure of a neuron includes the cell body, the dendrites, and the axons. The cell body, also called the soma, contains the nucleus. The nucleus contains the chromosomes. The dendrite of the neuron extends from the cell body and resembles the branches of a tree. The dendrite *receives* chemical messages from other cells across the synapse, a small gap. The axon is a thread-like extension of the cell body, which varies in length, up to 3 feet in the case of spinal nerves. The axon *transmits* an electro-chemical message along its length to another cell. Peripheral nervous system (PNS) neurons that deal with muscles are myelinated with fatty Schwann cell insulation to speed up the transmission of messages. Gaps between the Schwann cells that expose the axon are nodes of Ranvier and increase the speed of the transmission of nerve impulses along the axon. Neurons in the PNS that deal with pain are unmyelinated because transmission does not have to be as fast. Some neurons in the central nervous system (CNS) are myelinated by oligodendrocytes. If the myelin in the CNS oligodendrocytes breaks down, the patient develops multiple sclerosis (MS).

Urinary system

The principal function of the urinary system is to maintain the volume and composition of body fluids within normal limits. One aspect of this function is to rid the body of waste products that accumulate as a result of cellular metabolism, and because of this, it is sometimes referred to as the excretory system. The urinary system maintains an appropriate fluid volume by regulating the amount of water that is excreted in the urine.

Other aspects of its function include regulating the concentrations of various electrolytes in the body fluids and maintaining normal pH of the blood. In addition to maintaining fluid homeostasis in the body, the urinary system controls red blood cell production by secreting the hormone erythropoietin. The urinary system also plays a role in maintaining normal blood pressure by secreting the enzyme renin.

Structures of the Urinary System

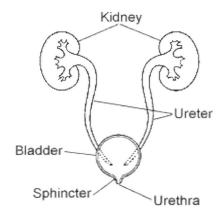

Integumentary system

The largest organ of the body is the skin. It forms the integumentary system, along with cutaneous glands, hair, and nails. The skin protects and cushions the body's delicate organs. Its functions are to:
- Excrete salts and nitrogenous wastes
- Metabolize Vitamin D
- Prevent bacteria, parasites, and other invaders from entering the body
- Protect the body from chemicals
- Produce melanin as sunscreen
- Protect the body from water loss
- Regulate body temperature through perspiration, fat storage, and radiating heat from capillaries
- Serve as sensory communication tool through temperature, touch, pain, and pressure receptors

It has three layers:
- The Epidermis - The epidermis, as its name suggests, is the outermost layer of the skin. It is comprised of four separate layers of epithelial tissue. The outermost layer of the epidermis is the stratum corneum. It is approximately 20-30 cells thick. The cells here are completely keratinized and dead, and this is what gives the skin its waterproof quality. The next two layers, the stratum granulosum and the stratum lucidum, are similar in that they represent an intermediate stage of keratinization. The cells here are not fully keratinized yet, but as the growth of the skin pushes them outward, they will increasingly move towards that state. The deepest layer of the epidermis is the stratum germinativum. The cells here are mitotically active-- that is, they are alive and reproducing. This is where the growth of skin takes place.

- The Dermis - The dermis is the second layer of skin, directly beneath the epidermis. Unlike the epidermis, the dermis has its own blood supply. Sweat glands are present to collect water and various wastes from the bloodstream, and excrete them through pores in the epidermis. The dermis is also the site of hair roots, and it is here where the growth of hair takes place. By the time hair reaches the environment outside of the skin, it has died. The dermis also contains dense connective tissue, made of collagen fibers, which gives the skin much of its elasticity and strength.
- The Subcutaneous Layer - Beneath the dermis lays the final layer of skin, the subcutaneous layer. The most notable structures here are the large groupings of adipose tissue. The main function of the subcutaneous layer is therefore to provide a cushion for the delicate organs lying beneath the skin. It also functions to insulate the body to maintain body temperature.

Skin can be damaged by chemicals, impact by sharp or blunt instruments, heat, friction, pressure and radiation. Among the injuries that can happen to the skin are abrasions, burns, contusions, crushing, decubitus ulcers (bedsores), gunshot, hematoma, incisions, lacerations, and punctures.

The following are the major structures found in skin:
- Pore- a tiny opening in the skin that serves as an outlet for sweat
- Sweat gland- any of the glands in the skin that secrete perspiration usually located in the dermis
- Nerve ending- the terminal structure of an axon that does not end at a synapse
- Erector pili- tiny smooth muscle fibers attached to each hair follicle, which contract to make the hairs stand on end
- Hair follicle- A hair follicle is part of the skin that grows hair by packing old cells together. Inside the follicle the sebaceous gland is found. At the end of the hair, tiny blood vessels form the root, around the root there is a white structure called a bulb, which is visible on plucked healthy hairs.
- Sebaceous gland- a gland in the skin that opens into a hair follicle and secretes an oily substance called sebum

Lymphatic system

The lymphatic system is the body's main protection against disease. The lymphatic system is comprised of the spleen, thymus, bone marrow, and a series of transparent tubes that run throughout the body, parallel to the blood vessels. The tubes are lymph vessels, and carry 4 liters of clear lymphatic fluid, or lymph. Lymph circulates throughout the body in the same manner as blood, with valves opening and closing to move the liquid along. There are about 100 small glands, called lymph nodes, stationed at intervals along the lymphatic vessels. The lymphatic fluid carries invaders to the nodes to be destroyed by lymphocytes, a type of white blood cell. Antibodies are also found in lymphatic fluid. Nodes swell during infections. Plasma from the blood vessels seeps out of the capillaries, immerses body tissues, and then drains off into the lymph vessels. Once in the lymphatic system, the plasma is called lymph. Lymph travels through the lymphatic vessels until it reaches the thoracic duct, the largest lymph vessel, extending from L2 to the neck. The lymph drains from the thoracic duct into the blood circulatory system.

Upper limb arteries

The arteries of the upper limb are as follows:
- Internal thoracic - Descends posterior to sternal end of clavicle and enters thorax
- Thyrocervical trunk- Ascends as short trunk, gives off four branches; transverse and ascending cervical, suprascapular
- Suprascapular - Passes inferolaterally, runs parallel to clavicle, then passes posteriorly to scapula
- Subscapular - Descends along lateral border of subscapularis to inferior angle of scapula
- Thoracodorsal - Accompanies thoracodorsal nerve to latissimus dorsi
- Deep Brachial - Accompanies radial nerve through radial groove in humerus, anastamoses around elbow joint
- Ulnar Collateral - Both anastamose around elbow joint

Blood

Blood has numerous functions – gas transport, haemostasis, defense against disease – all of which are brought about by its various components:
- Red blood cells – oxygen transport and gas exchange
- Blood platelets and coagulation factors – coagulation and haemostasis
- Vitamin K – essential cofactor in normal hepatic synthesis of some clotting factors
- Plasmin – lyses fibrin and fibrinogen
- Antithrombin III – inhibits IXa, Xa, XIa, XIIa,
- Complement – defense against pyogenic bacteria, activation of phagocytes, clearing of immune complexes, lytic attack on cell membranes
- Lymphocytes – adaptive immune response – killing of specific microbes
- Monocytes – respond to necrotic cell material by migrating to tissues and differentiating into macrophages
- Neutrophils – phagocytosis of microbes
- Eosinophils – phagocytosis, defense against helminthic parasites, allergic reactions
- Basophils – allergic reactions

Blood vessels

The types of blood vessels are:
- Arteries - blood vessels that carry blood away from the heart to the body, does not have valves
- Veins - blood vessels that carry the blood from the body back to the heart , has valves
- Capillaries – one cell thick blood vessels between arteries and veins that distribute oxygen-rich blood to the body
- Venules- the smallest veins
- Arterioles- the smallest arteries.

Layers of blood vessels
The wall of an artery consists of three (3) distinct layers of tunics:

- Tunica intima- Composed of simple, squamous epithelium called endothelium. Rests on a connective tissue membrane that is rich in elastic and collagenous fibers.
- Tunica media- Makes up the bulk of the arterial wall. Includes smooth muscle fibers, which encircle the tube, and a thick layer of elastic connective tissue.
- Tunica adventitia - Consists chiefly of connective tissue with irregularly arranged elastic and collagenous fibers. This layer attaches the artery to the surrounding tissues. Also contains minute vessels (vasa vasorum--vessels of vessels) that give rise to capillaries and provide blood to the more external cells of the artery wall.

Smooth muscles in the walls of arteries and arterioles are innervated by the sympathetic branches of the autonomic nervous system. The Tunica media and the Tunica adventitia are much thicker in arteries.

Forces that move blood through arteries vs. veins

The blood flowing through the arterial system is pushed by the pressure built up by the contractions of the heart. The blood flowing through the veins relies on skeletal muscle movement to keep the valves located in the veins opening and closing to keep blood moving towards the heart and not backwards through the system.

Pulse and blood pressure

Pulse is the expansion and contraction of a blood vessel due to the blood pumped through it; determined as the number of expansions per minute. Blood pressure is the force exerted in the arteries by blood as it circulates. It is divided into systolic (when the heart contracts) and diastolic (when the heart is filling) pressures.

Vascular system

The functions of the vascular system are as follows:
- Transport of materials:
    1. Gasses transported: Oxygen is transported from the lungs to the cells. CO_2 (a waste) is transported from the cells to the lungs.
    2. Transport other nutrients to cells - For example, glucose, a simple sugar used to produce ATP is transported throughout the body by the circulatory system. Immediately after digestion, glucose is transported to the liver. The liver maintains a constant level of glucose in the blood.
    3. Transport other wastes from cells - For example, ammonia is produced as a result of protein digestion. It is transported to the liver where it is converted to less toxic urea. Urea is then transported to the kidneys for excretion in the urine.
    4. Transport hormones - Numerous hormones that help maintain constant internal conditions are transported by the vascular system.
- Contains cells that fight infection
- Helps stabilize the pH and ionic concentration of the body fluids.
- It helps maintain body temperature by transporting heat.

Respiration

Internal respiration is the exchange of oxygen, carbon dioxide and trace gases at the cellular level. External respiration is the exchange of oxygen, carbon dioxide, and other gases between the lungs and blood, commonly known as breathing. The passage of gases through the respiratory system is as follows:

1. Inspiratory neurons in the respiratory center of the medulla oblongata (brain stem) tell the body to inhale
2. Nostrils and mouth warm inhaled air by moving it over nasal conchae and sinuses
3. Air passes through the pharynx to the larynx (voice box)
4. The epiglottis flips to cover the esophagus
5. Air passes into the trachea (windpipe)
6. Diaphragm contracts and flattens to raise the ribs as breathing occurs
7. Intercostal muscles between the ribs pull the ribs up enabling the chest to expand and air to pull inward
8. Trachea splits into the left and right bronchi that connect to the lungs. The bronchi split into fine branches called bronchioles
9. Bronchioles end in thin-walled, grape-like alveoli where the red blood cells absorb oxygen (O_2) from the inhaled air and give off carbon dioxide (CO_2).

Expiratory neurons in the brain stem tell the diaphragm and ribs to relax and exhale carbon dioxide into the atmosphere.

Arm nerves
The 4 key nerves of the arm are as follows:
- Musculocutaneous Nerve: Supplies all the muscles in the anterior (flexor) compartment of the arm. In the interval between the biceps and brachialis it becomes the lateral cutaneous nerve of forearm which supplies a large area of forearm skin.
- Radial Nerve: Supplies all the muscles in the posterior compartment of the arm, Descends inferolaterally with deep brachial artery around humerus in radial groove, Divides into deep and superficial branches: Deep Branch: entirely muscular in distribution, Superficial Branch: entirely cutaneous, supply dorsum of hand and digits.
- Median Nerve: No branches in arm. Runs initially on lateral side of brachial artery. Crosses it at middle of arm. Descends to cubital fossa deep to bicipital aponeurosis.
- Ulnar Nerve: No branches in arm. Passes anterior to triceps on medial side of brachial artery. Passes posterior to medial epicondyle and medial to olecranon to enter forearm.

Eyes

The following are the main parts of the eye and their functions:
- Aqueous humor is watery fluid that maintains eye pressure.
- The bony orbit is the socket protecting the eye.
- Cranial nerves that help with the function of the eye such as movement or vision include the optic nerve (cranial nerve II), oculomotor (III), trochlear (IV), trigeminal (V), abducens (VI), and vagus (X) nerves.
- Eyelashes and lids protect the eye and sweep out particles.

- Extrinsic muscles focus the eye.
- The lacrimal glands are tear ducts to moisten the eye.
- The lens refracts light.
- The optic disc is the blind spot.
- The pupil regulates light entry.
- The retina has rods for black and white imaging and cones for color imaging, and helps trigger the optic nerve to send impulses to the brain
- The macula is at the retinal center that is very sensitive to light.
- The black spot in the center is called the fovea which provides the sharpest vision.
- The choroid is a black layer behind the retina that absorbs light and nourishes the retina.
- The cornea is the window at the front of the eye that helps with focus.
- The iris regulates light entry
- The sclera is tough, white fibrous connective tissue holding nerves and vessels that acts as protection for the eye.
- The suspensory ligament connects the lens to the ciliary muscles of the iris.
- The vitreous humor is jelly that maintains the eye's shape and refracts images.

Anemia

Anemia refers to any condition where there is reduced oxygen carrying capacity due to a fall in hemoglobin concentration with resultant tissue hypoxia. It is defined as Hb less than 13.5g/dl in males, <11/5g/dl in females, <15g/dl in newborns to three month olds, and less than 11g/dl from three months to puberty. Anemia results when compensatory mechanisms fail to restore oxygen levels to meet tissue demands. The following compensatory mechanisms are seen – arteriolar dilatation, increased cardiac output, increased anaerobic metabolism, increased Hb dissociation, increased erythropoietin output, and internal redistribution of blood flow. If these compensatory mechanisms are adequate, oxygen levels are restored. If not, anemia ensues, with cardiac effects, poor exercise tolerance, lethargy, pallor, headaches, angina on effort and claudication.

Dysphagia

Esophageal dysphagia is difficulty swallowing. It is distinct from odynophagia, which is painful swallowing. Dysphagia can result from:
- Strictures, tumors or foreign bodies
- Motility disorders, including achalasia
- Spasms of the esophagus

Patients present with difficulty swallowing, choking or coughing during eating, chronic weight loss and aspiration pneumonia. The doctor diagnoses the cause of dysphagia with endoscopy, barium swallow and monometric studies of the esophagus. Patients with stroke, Parkinson's disease, multiple sclerosis, Lou Gehrig's disease, myasthenia gravis, muscular dystrophy, and various palsies are prone to dysphagia in their end stages. The treatment approach depends on the underlying cause of the dysphagia, and may include physiotherapy to retrain swallowing muscles, acid blocking medications, surgery to remove obstructions, or placement of a gastrostomy tube.

Alzheimer's disease

Alzheimer's disease is a degenerative disorder of the brain. It is the most common cause of dementia. It typically affects people 65 years of age and older, though early onset Alzheimer's disease can occur. The cause of Alzheimer's disease is unknown. Initial symptoms of Alzheimer's disease include loss of short-term memory or forgetfulness. As the disease progresses, the patient experiences increasing confusion and aggression, while losing long-term memory, language skills, and other cognitive functions. Death typically results from breakdown of bodily functions. Alzheimer's disease is incurable; management of the disease is the key to an extended life expectancy after diagnosis.

Dementia

Dementia is a term used to describe any cognitive dysfunction that may occur as a result of long-term illness, such as Alzheimer's disease, depression, and cerebral vascular accident. Dementia encompasses any resulting difficulties in memory, language, or problem-solving abilities. The patient is usually considered to be demented after six months of cognitive dysfunction; cognitive dysfunction that has gone on less than six months is typically referred to as delirium. Dementia may be curable, depending upon the cause. If the patient starts showing any signs of confusion, it should be reported to the nurse immediately.

There are a number of diseases and disorders that result in the onset of dementia. The most common cause of dementia is infection of the brain, such as meningitis or encephalitis. Both the infection and the resulting dementia typically resolve after treatment with antibiotics. Disorders that cause undue pressure on the brain, such as head injuries, hydrocephalus, and brain tumors, can cause dementia. There are treatments available to treat the increased pressure, and the dementia diminishes after the pressure has been relieved. Disorders that affect other body systems, such as liver disease, kidney disease, or pancreatic disease, can cause dementia by upsetting the delicate chemical balance within the body. In order to restore the patient's previous mental state, the chemical balance in the body must be restored.

Multi-infarct dementia is the second most common cause of irreversible cognitive dysfunction. It is caused by tissue damage that occurs when atherosclerotic plaque on the vessel wall breaks off and migrates to another part of the brain, where it creates a blockage. Because the brain tissue cannot get an adequate supply of blood flow, brain tissue in the area of the blockage dies from hypoxia. Though the blockages can be treated, cognitive function does not return after treatment. Huntington's disease is the degeneration of certain types of brain cells. Dementia often develops in the late stages of this disease.

Parkinson's disease

Parkinson's disease is a disorder that results in degeneration of the nervous system. It causes a decline in speech and motor skills and may cause a decline in cognitive function. Typical signs of Parkinson's disease include tremulousness, a shuffling gait, difficulty turning, difficulty speaking or swallowing, and a mask-like face. Parkinson's disease may also result in short-term memory loss and dementia in advanced cases. In most cases, the cause of Parkinson's disease is unknown, though in some cases the cause may be genetic or a result of a history of head trauma. Treatment includes medication management, management of symptoms, and surgery.

Sundowner's syndrome

Sundowner's syndrome is a condition in which patients become increasingly confused in the late afternoon or early evening. It is most commonly seen in patients with a history of Alzheimer's disease or dementia; however, it can occur in patients who do not have a history of dementia. Though a number of theories exist as to why Sundowner's syndrome occurs, the actual cause is unknown. Patients who are suffering from Sundowner's syndrome may experience worsening confusion, restlessness, or agitation. Some patients may experience hallucinations or wandering as part of Sundowner's syndrome.

Aphasia

Aphasia is defined as difficulty speaking that results from lesions on the brain. Aphasia is typically caused by cerebral vascular accident, brain injury, brain tumors, or by progressive diseases, such as Alzheimer's disease or Parkinson's disease. Aphasia can come in a number of different forms. The patient may be unable to speak or may speak using inappropriate words and phrases. The patient may become unable to name objects or call objects by the wrong names. Aphasia can also affect the patient's ability to comprehend language. With aphasia, the patient may become unable to read, write, or form complete sentences.

Mental changes involved in aging

Cognitive impairment in the elderly typically becomes noticeable at around 60 years of age, though the rate of decline varies depending on the individual. As a person ages, he typically experiences a mild decline in the ability to retrieve words and name common objects. Memory also tends to decline as a person ages. The ability to encode new information declines, typically as a result of a decline in sensory abilities. Short-term memory may also decline, though significant changes in long-term memory are typically not seen until about 70 to 80 years of age. The rate of memory decline can be stemmed using memory exercises and problem-solving skills.

Depression

Depression is a disorder in which the patient experiences a consistently low mood, coupled with feelings of worthlessness, sadness, or self-loathing. The patient may experience insomnia (inability to sleep) or hypersomnia (sleeping too much). The patient may also complain of digestive difficulties or frequent headaches. Severe cases of depression may result in increased forgetfulness or hallucinations. Depression can be caused by a number of physical, psychological, or sociological factors. Physical characteristics, such as a small hippocampus of the brain, may lead to the onset of depression. Depression may also be brought on by life-altering illnesses, such as Parkinson's disease, heart attack, or stroke. Tragic life events and the inability to effectively cope with them may also lead to an onset of depression.

Burns

The ER physician classifies burns by the Rule of Nines. You will hear the Rule of Nines when transcribing:

- In an adult, each part of the body contributes the following percentage to the entire body surface area: Perineum, 1%; each leg, 18%; each arm, 9%; chest and abdomen, 18%; back and buttocks, 18%; and head, 9%.
- In a child, each part of the body contributes the following percentage to the entire body surface area: Each leg, 16%; each arm, 9%; chest and abdomen, 18%; back and buttocks, 18%; and head, 14%.
- In an infant, each part of the body contributes the following percentage to the entire body surface area: Each leg, 14%; each arm, 9%; chest and abdomen, 18%, back and buttocks, 18%, and head, 18%. The palm of the hand and groin are *each* 1% of the entire body surface.
- The ER doctor uses the Rule of Nines to determine when to give fluid resuscitation (20—25%) and when to transfer the patient to the Burn Unit. Burns to the face and palms are usually critical.

Diabetic coma and diabetic shock

Diabetic coma results from prolonged high blood sugar (hyperglycemia) caused by too much sugar or carbohydrates and not enough insulin. Initially, the patient's mental status alters. He/she is confused, thirsty, and exhibits drunken behavior. The patient urinates frequently and may vomit. He/she complains of nausea and abdominal pain. The skin is flushed and dry. The patient snores when he/she eventually sinks into coma. Ketones will be present in the urine, the blood sugar level will be elevated and the patient's breath may have a fruity odor. Stop the procedure. The patient will require insulin. Fluid replacement is required. Inform the doctor.

Diabetic shock is also known as insulin shock and results from sudden low blood sugar (hypoglycemia, glucose less than 70 mg/dl) through fasting, overexertion, alcohol ingestion, stress, or drug reactions. The patient displays nervousness, irritability, shaking, cold sweats, and complains of hunger. Loss of consciousness follows. Stop the procedure. The rule of 15 should be followed where 15 grams of carbohydrate is given then the blood glucose can be rechecked in 15 minutes. Give 4 ounces of orange juice, or a glucose drink, or 3-4 glucose tablets, or 6-8 Lifesavers candies immediately. A delay may cause your patient to become unresponsive and require glucagon injections, or hospital treatment for acidosis. If the blood glucose is still low after 15 minutes, the procedure should be repeated.

Fracture

A fracture is a break or disruption in the integrity of a bone that occurs when force or weight are applied to the bone, which exceed the bone's ability to remain structurally intact. Fractures occur from direct or indirect trauma, or because of diseases (e.g., cancer and osteoporosis) and congenital states such as contractures. Fractures are frequently associated with adjacent soft tissue injuries. Modern fractures are classified as either open or closed. Older fracture classifications still used in transcriptions include:
- Simple (skin intact, no bone contact with air); compound (bone protrudes through skin)
- Comminuted (splintered)
- Compacted (bone ends are jammed together)
- Spiral (twisted, as in a skiing accident)
- Compression (where the patient loses height because the spine fuses)

- Oblique (diagonal to the axis); transverse (right angled to the axis)
- Linear (parallel to the axis)
- Incomplete (bone is still joined at some points)
- Complete (bone fragments are completely separated)
- Greenstick (twisted immature bones)

Epilepsy, absence, and tonic/clonic seizures

Epilepsy is an electric storm in the brain from uncontrolled, synchronized firing of neurons. Epilepsy can be acquired from head injury or innate, from neural membranes abnormally permeable to sodium and potassium. Anticonvulsants like Tegretol, phenobarb and Dilantin control epilepsy. An absence is a generalized seizure, formerly called petit mal, with no specific focus in the brain. The patient stares, lip smacks, and blinks for a few seconds. Absences begin and end without warning and are difficult to discern because there is no after-effect. However, a 3 Hz spike and wave discharges result on an EEG. Absence seizures interfere with learning. The patient is unaware of what occurred during the seizure. Youths 7—19 are prone to seizures from flashing strobe lights at discos and flickering TV patterns. A famous case is the December 1997 Pokémon episode that sent 700 children to hospital; 500 had confirmed seizures. Tonic-clonic seizure (grand mal) is a convulsion involving the entire brain. An aura may precede the seizure (smell, lights, or other warning symptom). Muscles contract during tonic phase, breathing is irregular, and skin is blue tinged from lack of oxygen (cyanosis). The patient loses bladder control. In clonic phase, limbs jerk from quick muscle contraction and relaxation. After the seizure, the patient is limp, regains consciousness gradually, and is confused. Recovery takes hours.

Signs and treatment of stroke

Signs and symptoms of stroke (cerebrovascular accident or CVA) include: Disruptions in vision; trouble speaking or expressing thoughts; headache; weakness affecting one side of the body; difficulty walking; and numbness or tingling on one side of the body. Loss of consciousness is rare. The patient may be having a transient ischemic attack (TIA or mini-stroke), which is a warning of an impending stroke. Give the patient 2 Aspirins and call EMS (911). Place the patient in recovery position with the affected side down, the head slightly elevated, and cover him/her with a blanket. Bring the crash cart. Paramedics will ask the patient to smile, to extend the arms for 10 seconds with the eyes closed, and to repeat a phrase. The base hospital doctor may order the paramedics to administer dipyridamole (Persantine), clopidogrel (Plavix), or ticlopidine (Ticlid). Approximately 33% of patients who experience a transient ischemic attack will have recurrent attacks. Complete stroke (CVA) is diagnosed if neurological signs and symptoms last more than 24 hours. It is imperative to obtain medical care as soon as possible to improve outcome. Tissue Plasminogen Activator (tPA) should be started immediately if appropriate. It can only be given within 3 hours of symptoms starting to reduce the chance for long term disability. Approximately 5% of patients who have a transient ischemic attack will have a cerebrovascular accident within one month, and 30% of will have a cerebrovascular accident within one year.

Wounds

The different types of wounds and their proper treatment are as follows:

- Contusion - A raised bruise (hematoma). Treat contusions during the first 48 hours by applying cold packs for 15 minutes on and 15 minutes off, taking acetaminophen or ibuprofen, and elevating the area. Warm washcloths help after the second day.
- Laceration - A long break in the surface of the skin. The edges of a laceration may be linear (smooth) or stellate (irregular). A laceration is caused by a knife blow, glass, or a surgeon's scalpel and usually requires sutures.
- Abrasion - A scrape or scratch of the outer layer of the skin. Friction burns and rug burns are types of abrasions. Wash the wound and remove gravel with a forceps.
- Avulsion - A flap of tissue that is torn away from the main body of tissue, which often requires sutures.
- Puncture - A small, deep perforation of the skin caused by teeth, needles, ice-picks, small caliber bullets, and other narrow, sharp objects. The doctor irrigates and probes the puncture.
- Amputation - The body part is completely detached. Wrap the amputated part in a sterile dressing and place in a labeled plastic bag on ice. A surgeon may be able to reattach it.

Dehydration

Dehydration is a life-threatening condition that occurs when the body does not have enough water to perform normal body functions. Patients who are dehydrated may present with sunken eyes and dry mucous membranes. Dehydrated patients will often complain of generalized weakness and constant thirst. Their skin may lose its elasticity as a result of dehydration. They may have a weak, rapid pulse and a low blood pressure. The urine will become darker and more concentrated when patients are dehydrated; a result of the kidneys conserving as much water as possible. Dehydration can be caused by too little intake or too much output. Limited intake may result if the patient is unable to take in fluid as a result of chronic nausea or difficulty swallowing. The patient may be unable to obtain an adequate amount of fluid if he is confused or kept NPO. Dehydration may also result if the patient is excreting too much fluid. The most common cause of over-excretion of fluid is frequent diarrhea. Excessive sweating from fever or exercise may also result in excessive fluid loss. Blood loss after surgery or a hemorrhage or fluid loss after a burn may also cause dehydration.

Fluid overload

If a patient is suspected to be in fluid overload, he should be monitored closely. The most significant sign of fluid overload is increased respiratory distress or crackles in the bases of the lungs. The patient may experience edema in the extremities, puffiness around the eyes, or fluid accumulation (ascites) in the abdomen. As the fluid accumulates, the patient may have an unexplained weight gain over a short period of time. A patient in fluid overload may have a bounding pulse, hypertension, or bulging veins. If any of these signs are noticed, the nurse should be notified immediately. Fluid overload can be caused by excessive fluid intake or by previous medical conditions. Excessive fluid intake can occur if the patient is receiving too much IV fluid or is taking in too much oral intake. The patient's intake and output balance should be closely monitored to ensure the patient does not continue to take in too much fluid. Sodium intake should be monitored as well as too much salt may cause an increased fluid absorption by the kidneys, resulting in fluid overload. Certain medical conditions, such as heart attack or heart failure, place the patient at an increased risk of fluid overload as the heart may not be able to accommodate an increased amount of fluid. Patients with a history of kidney failure may not be able to effectively compensate for fluid overload and should be closely monitored.

Constipation and diarrhea

Constipation occurs when the patient's stool is too dry and hard to be able to be passed easily, making him unable to have a bowel movement. The feces become dry and hard as a result of too much water being absorbed from the stool due to poor gastrointestinal motility. If the constipation is not treated, the patient may develop a bowel obstruction. Diarrhea refers to the frequent passage of loose or watery stools. Diarrhea places the patient at risk for developing dehydration because of the amount of fluid lost with the stool. Electrolytes are passed along with the fluid, which can lead to life-threatening electrolyte imbalances if not properly corrected.

Urinary tract infection

The primary symptom of a urinary tract infection is painful or difficult urination. The patient may exhibit cloudy urine, which may have a strong or foul smell. The patient may experience the need to urinate frequently or may have sudden urgency in the need to urinate. The patient may also complain of flank pain or pressure in the pelvis. The patient may show signs of a generalized infection, such as an elevated temperature, flushed skin, or malaise. An elderly patient may also show signs of confusion as a result of the infection.

DVT

A DVT, or deep vein thrombosis, is a blood clot that develops in the larger veins in an extremity. DVTs most commonly form in the legs, though the risk of developing a DVT in the arms does increase if the patient has an intravenous line. DVTs are most commonly caused by immobilization, though other factors such as obesity, infection, tobacco use, and advanced age can increase the patient's risk for developing a clot. The most common signs of a DVT include swelling and redness of the affected extremity. The patient may also complain of pain in the affected extremity.

Pressure sore stages

Pressure sores are divided into four stages, classified by the depth of the wound. A Stage I pressure sore refers to an area of redness that is typically located over a bony prominence. The reddened area may feel painful or warm to the touch. A Stage II pressure sore refers to wearing away of the first layer of skin, revealing a pink wound bed below. A Stage III pressure sore extends past the full thickness of the skin; fatty tissue may be visualized. Tunneling may also be present. A Stage IV pressure sore is the most severe, referring to a loss of enough skin tissue to reveal muscle tissue or bone.

Important terms

- Arrhythmia-An abnormal rate of muscle contractions in the heart which can present as bradycardia(too slow), tachycardia (too fast) or irregular
- Cervix- The neck of the womb located at the top of the vagina

- Extrasystole- A premature systole resulting in a momentary cardiac arrhythmia referred to as an extra heart beat
- Fallopian tubes- Two thin tubes that extend from each side of the uterus, toward the ovaries, as a passageway for eggs and sperm
- Fibrillation- Rapid, inefficient contraction of muscle fibers of the heart caused by disruption of nerve impulses
- Frontal (Coronal) plane - A plane parallel to the long axis of the body and perpendicular to the sagittal plane that separates the body into front and back portions.
- Murmur- The noise between normal heart sounds caused by blood flow through a heart valve
- Ova- A female sex cell, or egg
- Ovaries- The female sex gland with both a reproductive function (releasing ova) and a hormonal function (production of estrogen and progesterone)
- Sagittal plane - A plane that divides the body into right and left halves
- Transverse (Horizontal) plane - A plane that divides the body into upper and lower sections
- Uterus- The hollow female reproductive organ in which a fertilized egg is implanted and a fetus develops also known as the womb

Infection Control

Chain of infection

Chain of infection

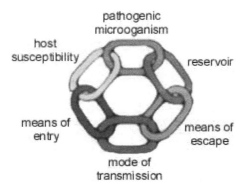

Risk for infection from patient care equipment

The level of risk for infection refers to the likelihood that a piece of equipment will contain infectious pathogens on its surface; it aids in determining the proper level of cleaning prior to subsequent use:

- Low-risk or noncritical items are pieces of equipment that come into contact with intact skin, such as stethoscopes. Noncritical items also include inanimate objects in the environment, such as countertops and walls. These items only require cleaning with a detergent prior to subsequent use.
- Intermediate-risk items are those that come in close contact with mucous membranes but do not penetrate the skin, such as thermometers or respiratory equipment. These items require cleaning with a high-level disinfectant before they are ready for use.
- High-risk items, such as surgical instruments and devices, have penetrated the skin and are at high risk for contamination by microorganisms. These items require sterilization before they are ready for subsequent use.

Bacterial and viral infection

A bacterial infection is caused when bacteria are introduced into the body. The bacteria multiply to infect the patient, resulting in infection. Bacterial infection is typically localized. For example, a throat infection may result in worse pain on one side of the throat. Antibiotics can be prescribed to help kill bacterial growth. Viral infections occur when a virus invades through the mucous membranes. It attaches itself to a living cell and uses its genetic material to produce more of the virus. This results in the death of the host cell. Viral infections do not respond to antibiotic treatment. Though some antiviral medications exist, the usual course of treatment in a viral infection is to treat the symptoms and bolster the immune system to fight the infection.

- 64 -

Signs and symptoms of infection

Infections are divided into two groups, localized and systemic. A localized infection occurs when a virus or bacteria begins to grow in a small area of the body. This can occur in wounds or surgical sites if not treated properly. Signs and symptoms of a localized infection include warmth, redness, and swelling around the site; purulent or foul-smelling drainage; or a fever. In a systemic infection, a virus or bacteria has gained access to the bloodstream, spreading to other parts of the body as a result. Signs of a systemic infection include fever, malaise, nausea, vomiting, chills, and generalized weakness.

Transmission of microorganisms

Microorganisms must move from one host to another in order to survive. Some microorganisms are transmitted via droplets that are released when an infected host coughs or sneezes. The microorganisms in the droplets can then invade a new host via the mucous membranes of the eyes, nose, or mouth. Microorganisms may also be transmitted through direct oral contact, such as through kissing an infected person or by drinking from the same cup as the sick individual. Iatrogenic transmission occurs when microorganisms move to a new host during a medical procedure, such as a surgery or line placement. On rare occasions, microorganisms can be transmitted through the fecal-oral route. This most typically occurs as a result of indirect contact with fecal material, such as through poor hand washing or by eating foods that have been contaminated.

Routes biological hazards may enter the body

The following are the routes that biological hazards may take to enter the body:
- Airborne (through the nasal passage into the lungs)
- Ingestion (by eating)
- Broken Skin
- Percutaneous (through intact skin)
- Mucosal (through the lining of the mouth and nose)

Infection control methods

The first line of defense in infection control is hand washing. Protective Clothing is an important aspect of infection control. This includes Masks, Goggles, Face Shields, Respirators, Gowns, Lab Coats, and Gloves. The precautions that are used depend on the infection. Isolation procedures are also used this includes protective isolation or reverse isolation. In protective isolation, the patients are isolated to prevent them from getting an infection i.e. patients receiving chemotherapy. In reverse isolation, the patients are isolated to prevent others from getting their infection or disease i.e. patients with tuberculosis. Universal Precautions are used with all patients. This means do not touch or use anything that has the patient's body fluid on it without a barrier and assume that all body fluid of a patient is infectious.

Hand washing

Microorganisms are present on all surfaces and can be transferred via touch. Certain microorganisms can cause illness or infection if they come into contact with a person whose immune system has been compromised. As a result, hand washing is a vital part of infection control. If properly done, hand washing removes visible dirt and germs from the hands. It prevents transmission of germs from the patient care technician to the patient or from one patient to another patient. Warm water, antimicrobial soap, and firm friction applied to all areas of the hand while washing are all key factors in ensuring that the hands are clean and free of germs.

Hand washing should be performed frequently to prevent transmission of germs. The patient care technician should wash her hands prior to eating, after going to the bathroom, or after sneezing. The patient care technician should also wash her hands prior to feeding the patient, before performing any procedures with the patient, and after the procedure is complete. Hand washing should be performed after coming into contact with a patient's wound, with soiled linen, or with any patient body fluids, even if the patient care technician was wearing gloves at the time. The patient care technician should also wash her hands prior to leaving the patient's room.

Before beginning to wash, remove any jewelry on your hands. Use clean, dry paper towels to turn on the taps. Run the water until it is warm, and then wet hands to the wrist. Apply disinfectant soap (poviodine scrub or bar soap rinsed and stored in a drainer). Continue to work the soap into a lather for at least 30 seconds, using firm friction between the fingers, underneath the fingernails, and up the wrists. Make sure to keep your hands lower than the elbows to prevent germs from traveling up the arm. If your hands have been soiled with body fluids, hand washing should be performed for at least one minute. Rinse hands thoroughly with warm water, and then dry your hands. When your hands are dry, use part of the towel to turn the faucet off. Note any cuts, rashes, broken or long nails that need treatment before resuming work.

Proper hand washing is the key to infection control. Because germs run off the hands while hand washing is performed, it is important to ensure that hands do not touch the inside of the sink while washing. If a patient care technician's hands touch the inside of the sink, then hand washing should be repeated to ensure her hands have not become contaminated. The wet surface of bar soap can provide a medium for germs to grow. Prior to beginning to wash hands, rub the soap vigorously to remove the outermost layer of soap. Then, once hand washing has been completed, rinse the soap with warm water.

If there is no sink nearby, use 70% to 80% alcohol cleanser (Cutan, Florafree, Manorapid, Purell) for 15 seconds, followed by disposable antiseptic towelettes (benzalkonium chloride). Change gloves frequently by turning them inside out from the wrists. Wash your hands as soon as possible.

Alcohol scrub

Hand sanitizers have been approved as an adjunct to hand washing in the health care setting. They work by removing the outer layer of oils on the hand, killing any bacteria on the hand in the process. To use alcohol scrub, take a dime-sized amount into your dominant hand. Rub your hands together vigorously for at least thirty seconds. Make sure to rub between your fingers, between your knuckles, and beneath the fingernails. If, after thirty seconds, your hands are still damp, allow them to air dry. Once your hands have dried, they are considered clean.

Though hand sanitizer has been approved as an adjunct for hand washing, it was not intended to replace it. There are instances in which hand washing is preferred over use of an alcohol-based hand sanitizer. A patient care technician should wash her hands if they have been soiled with secretions. Hand washing should be used prior to eating and after using the bathroom. Even if hand sanitizer is used, hands should occasionally be washed to remove any residue that can build up as a result of frequent use of alcohol scrub.

Isolation

Isolation refers to special measures taken to prevent the spread of germs. The goal is to protect other patients and hospital staff while providing care to the patient. Isolation may be required if the patient has a particularly infectious disease, such as tuberculosis or Varicella. The patient may also be placed into isolation if he has a drug-resistant bacterium, such as methicillin-resistant staphylococcus aureus (MRSA) or clostridium difficile (C. diff). Depending upon the type of isolation, the patient care technician may be required to wear an isolation gown, gloves, or a mask while providing care for the patient.

There are three types of isolation. Contact precautions are intended to limit the spread of microorganisms that might be transmitted by direct contact with a contaminated surface. If a patient is in contact isolation, he should be in a private room that is clearly marked. When providing care to the patient, the patient care technician should wear an isolation gown and gloves at all times while in the room. Droplet precautions are intended to limit the spread of microorganisms that are transmitted via mucous or respiratory secretions. A patient who requires droplet precautions should be placed in a private room. A patient care technician should wear a mask and gloves when caring for a patient who is in droplet precautions. Airborne precautions are intended to prevent the spread of airborne microorganisms that can survive for long periods of time in the environment. While on airborne precautions, the patient should be placed in a negative pressure room. While caring for the patient, the patient care technician should wear a mask or respirator and gloves.

The patient care technician should take care to ensure that germs from a patient in isolation are not spread amid the patient population. A cart should be placed outside of the patient's room containing isolation equipment that should be donned prior to entering the room. This includes waterproof isolation gowns, gloves, and masks, as well as a garbage bag for waste disposal. Germicidal wipes should also be available to clean the equipment that must be shared with the rest of the patient population. The patient in isolation can also be provided with disposable equipment that might ordinarily be shared among the patient population, such as single-use stethoscopes and blood pressure cuffs.

Isolation equipment should be donned before entering an isolation room. The gown should be unfolded and held with the opening toward your back. Place your arms through the sleeves. Tie the gown securely behind the neck and at the waist. Then, put on the facemask, making sure your nose and mouth are covered. Gloves should be applied last and worn so they cover the cuffs of the isolation gown. Isolation gear should be removed prior to leaving the room. The gloves should be removed first. Grasp the first glove at the wrist and pull to remove it. Then ball the used glove in the hand that is still gloved. Grasp the remaining glove at the wrist and pull to remove it. Next, remove the gown and the mask. Once the gloves, gown, and mask have been removed, wash your hands.

<u>Removal of soiled linen</u>
Care must be taken while removing soiled linen from an isolation room. Because the linen bag was in the isolation room, it is considered contaminated. The soiled linen bag must be placed inside a clean bag to prevent contamination. While the patient care technician is bathing the patient, soiled linen should be placed in a plastic linen bag. Once bathing has been completed, the linen bag should be tied securely shut. Another aide standing outside the door should hold a second linen bag open while the first bag is placed inside; the second bag should also be tied securely shut. The double-bagged linen bag should be left outside while the patient care technician removes her isolation gown, gloves, and mask, and washes her hands. Then, the soiled linen can be taken to the soiled utility room.

Medical asepsis

Medical asepsis means controlling the spread of hospital-acquired (nosocomial) disease and cross-infections (different pathogens passed between two patients):
- Wash your hands for 20-30 seconds using warm water and soap, taking care to clean your fingernails thoroughly whenever visibly soiled, before and after any contact with patients, and after gloves are removed
- Disinfect patient care materials before use with the proper chemical agent, according to the manufacturer's specifications
- Maintain a clean patient care environment, with adequate space, ventilation, sunlight, and cool temperature
- Dispose of infectious material as soon as soiling is discovered in the proper bin (concurrent cleaning)
- Disinfect patient care materials after a patient leaves the office, or dies, or is transferred to another floor or facility (terminal cleaning)
- Use Clean and Dirty Utility Rooms to separate unused equipment from used equipment and prevent contamination
- Store clean linen separate from used linen and limit access to the Clean Linen Room to authorized personnel only

Surgical asepsis

Surgical asepsis means sterilizing instruments, sutures, drapes, sponges, and other equipment used for surgery and storing them safely, so they do not become reinfected. Surgical equipment pierces the skin or mucous membranes, or is placed inside a wound, or is inserted into a body cavity that is normally sterile. Sterility is not required for instruments introduced into the vagina, ear canal, or mouth; a vaginal speculum, otoscope, or tongue depressor can be clean (disinfected), rather than sterile. Surgical equipment must be free of all microorganisms, including spores. Clean the field where you will sterilize the instruments. Wash your hands thoroughly for 2-5 minutes using an antimicrobial soap then glove. Use sterile supplies only. After you sterilize the instruments in an autoclave pack, create a sterile field. Find a clean, flat, dry surface that is free from drafts. Wash your hands and don sterile gloves. Cover the field with a sterile drape. Open the autoclave pack on the drape. Keep sterile all articles that touch the sterile field.

Cleaning, disinfection, and sterilization

Cleaning refers to the process that removes visible dirt or soiled material from a surface. It typically involves using water or a detergent to rinse the surface. Cleaning must be performed prior to disinfection or sterilization. Disinfection is defined as the process that destroys most microorganisms on the surface of a piece of equipment. The disinfectant that is used is typically chemical in nature, though some pieces of equipment may be disinfected using heat. Sterilization refers to the process that removes all forms of microbial life from a piece of equipment.

Sterilization
Sterilization requires a piece of equipment be exposed to extreme dry heat or a chemical sterilant to remove all microorganisms. Equipment is typically exposed to dry heat during the autoclaving process. Autoclaving is considered to be the most effective method of sterilization. Chemical sterilization is used for equipment unable to tolerate high temperatures, such as fluids and rubber. Care must be taken when handling sterile equipment. Any contact with a non-sterile surface will introduce new microorganisms to the equipment. When a piece of sterile equipment is prepared for use, it should be handled using sterile technique.

Cleaning
Cleaning refers to the process of removing dirt or organic material from the surface of a piece of equipment. If an item is not properly cleaned, subsequent disinfection or sterilization may not be effective. Gloves should be worn while cleaning equipment. Thoroughly wipe each piece of equipment with a detergent, rubbing with firm pressure to remove any dirt or organic material. Once the organic material and dirt has been removed, rinse the surface thoroughly with water and allow it to dry prior to subsequent use. Hand washing should be performed after cleaning any equipment.

Universal precautions

Universal precautions involve treating all patient secretions as if they contain a pathogen, resulting in the avoidance of direct contact with any secretions. Universal precautions are practiced in the health care setting whenever there is the risk of coming into contact with blood or body fluids. The precautions include wearing gloves when collecting blood or handling anything that may have been contaminated with blood. Use of other protective equipment may be necessary, such as wearing a face shield when suctioning copious secretions or a facemask to protect oneself from airborne secretions. If blood or body fluids have contaminated a work surface, it should be cleaned using the appropriate disinfectant.

Personal protective equipment

Gloves are the most commonly used piece of protective equipment in the health care setting. They are typically made of thin vinyl or nitrile rubber and are intended for single use. They should be used whenever there is a risk of touching infectious material or body fluids. Gowns are typically made of thin plastic or synthetic waterproof fibers. They are typically worn over the uniform whenever the patient is in contact isolation. Face protection falls into two categories. Facemasks are worn over the nose and mouth to prevent inhalation of infectious material. Goggles are worn over the eyes to prevent introduction of infectious materials to the eyes. When dealing with a copious amount of secretions, a face shield can be worn in place of a facemask and goggles.

Changing linens

While removing dirty linens, the patient care technician should wear gloves and avoid holding them close to her body. Soiled linens should not be shaken out as this may release germs into the air. Once all of the soiled linens have been removed from the bed and put into the appropriate receptacle, the patient care technician should remove her gloves and wash her hands. She should then securely tie the linen bag closed and place it in the soiled utility room. Clean linens should be carefully unfolded and placed on the bed. Any linen that has fallen on the floor should be considered contaminated; it should be placed in the soiled utility bin and replaced with clean linen.

Hepatitis B virus

Hepatitis B is a sexually transmitted disease also transmitted with body fluids, and some individuals may be symptom free but still be carriers. Condoms are not proved to prevent the spread of this disease. Symptoms include:
- Jaundice
- Dark Urine
- Malaise
- Joint pain
- Fever
- Fatigue

Tests include:
- Decreased albumin levels, + antibodies and antigen
- Increased levels of transaminase

Treatment includes:
- Monitor for changes in the liver.
- Recombinant alpha interferon in some cases.
- Transplant necessary if liver failure occurs.

Prevention:
Series of 3 Hepatitis B Vaccinations: an initial dose, a dose 1 month later and a final dose 6 months after the initial dose.

HBV is the most common laboratory-associated infection.

Hepatitis D virus

Hepatitis D is usually acquired with HBV as a co-infection or super infection. Signs and symptoms include jaundice, fatigue, abdominal pain, loss of appetite, nausea, vomiting, joint pain, and dark (tea colored) urine. Transmission occurs when blood from an infected person enters the body of a person who is not immune by sharing drugs, needles, or "works" when "shooting" drugs; through needle sticks or sharps exposures on the job; or from an infected mother to her baby during birth.

Treatment includes:
- Acute HDV infection - Supportive care
- Chronic HDV infection interferon-alfa, liver transplant

Prevention includes:
- Hepatitis B vaccination
- HBV-HDV co-infection: pre- or post-exposure prophylaxis (hepatitis B immune globulin or vaccine) to prevent HBV infection
- HBV-HDV superinfection: education to reduce risk behaviors among persons with chronic HBV infection

HIV transmission

HIV can be transmitted from an infected person to an uninfected one in the following ways:
- Unprotected sexual contact. Direct blood contact, including injection drug needles, blood transfusions, accidents in health care settings or certain blood products. Mother to baby (before or during birth, or through breast milk)
- Sexual intercourse (vaginal and anal): In the genitals and the rectum, HIV may infect the mucous membranes directly or enter through cuts and sores caused during intercourse (many of which would be unnoticed).
- Oral sex (mouth-penis, mouth-vagina): The mouth is an inhospitable environment for HIV (in semen, vaginal fluid or blood), meaning the risk of HIV transmission through the throat, gums, and oral membranes is lower than through vaginal or anal membranes. There are however, documented cases where HIV was transmitted orally. Sharing injection needles: An injection needle can pass blood directly from one person's bloodstream to another. It is a very efficient way to transmit a blood-borne virus.
- Mother to Child: It is possible for an HIV-infected mother to pass the virus directly before or during birth, or through breast milk. The following "bodily fluids" are NOT infectious: saliva, tears, sweat, feces, and urine

Small blood spills

The best way to clean a small blood spill is to absorb the blood with a paper towel or gauze pad. Then disinfect area with a disinfectant. Soap and water is not a disinfectant nor is alcohol. Never scrape a dry spill; this may cause an aerosol of infectious organisms. If blood is dried, use the disinfectant to moisten the dried blood.

Disposal of biohazardous material

Wear a gown, gloves, and mask when handling all tissue. Post biohazard signs on walls and containers. Properly label all containers. Ventilate biohazardous areas very well; consult your Safety Officer regarding fume hoods and filters. Avoid using aerosols, especially for quick freezing tissue, because they increase your risk of exposure to infectious material. Dispose of all soft waste material in red or yellow biohazard bags, and disposable blades in red or yellow sharps containers. Disinfect non-disposable objects, such as tables. The CDC and EPA recommend steam sterilization and incineration for all waste except pathological waste, which only needs incineration. Dispose of blood in the sink with adequately running water. If you or a co-worker is exposed to hazardous materials, start decontamination procedures immediately. Check the written procedures in your policy and procedures manual (P&P). By law, P&Ps must be readily available to all staff, and your employer must train staff fully to use them.

Biohazard symbol

Biohazard symbol

Protective clothing

A healthcare worker puts on the protective gown first being sure not to touch the outside of the gown. The mask is put on next. Gloves are applied last and secured over the cuffs of the gown. A healthcare worker removes the gloves first. They are removed by grasping one glove at the wrist and pulling it inside out off the hand and holding it in the gloved hand. The second glove is removed by placing your uncovered hands fingers under the edge of the glove being careful not to touch the outside of the glove and rolling it down inside out over the glove grasped in your hand. The first glove ends up inside of the second glove. Next, remove your mask by touching the strings only. Next slide your arms out of the gown and then fold the gown with the outside folded in away from your body so that the contaminated side is folded inwardly. Dispose of properly. Always wash hands after glove removal.

Important terms

- Antisepsis - Antisepsis is reducing the flora and transient microorganisms on the skin for minor procedures like venipuncture. Clean gloves are worn. It requires a short-acting antiseptic like 70% isopropyl alcohol that can denature proteins.
- Asepsis - Asepsis prevents infection during surgical procedures by reducing pathogens. It requires sterile instruments and sterile gloves, and a strong disinfectant that can kill both Gram-positive and Gram-negative bacteria and their resistant spores, like 70% povidone-iodine.
- Communicable infection - An illness due to a specific infectious agent or its toxic products that arises through transmission of that agent or its products from an infected person, animal or inanimate reservoir to a susceptible host; either directly or indirectly through an intermediate plant or animal host, vector or the inanimate environment (synonym: infectious disease)
- Modified isolation - Modified isolation attempts to limit infection with protective techniques, like donning gloves, gowns, and masks when handling the patient's body fluids. Reverse isolation - Reverse isolation protects a patient from others in a clean room, as after kidney transplant.
- Nosocomial infection - Illnesses acquired in the hospital inpatient environment not resulting from the reasons the patient was admitted

- Standard/universal precautions - Standard or universal precautions means healthcare workers control the spread of disease by assuming every patient's samples are infectious, and following the U.S. Occupational Safety and Health Administration (OSHA) standards for proper hand washing, wearing gloves and other personal protective equipment , bagging specimens in biohazard bags, and disposing of needles and lancets in a sharps safe.
- Strict isolation - Strict isolation segregates infectious patients to one room, and visitors are restricted.

Phlebotomy and Related Procedures

Initiating patient contact

The steps in initiating patient contact are as follows:
1. Knock on door before entering patient's room, slowly open the door and ask if it is alright to enter.
2. Look for signs on door indicating special precautions that you need to take i.e. protective clothing needed
3. Identify your name and reason for entering room
4. In the event of a Physician or Member of the Clergy being in the room, it is not inappropriate to explain who you are and proceed to do the draw if the draw is STAT.
5. Ask the family to step out of the room.

Proper patient identification

Proper patient identification is important because it can prevent a critical error like misidentifying a patient specimen which could result in harm or death to a patient. Patient identification includes asking a patient to state their name and date of birth, and then you check the identification band and the requisition to see if they match. Verbal identification should never be relied on alone although it is important since patients can be hard of hearing, ill, or mentally incompetent and may give incorrect information. Also, check the identification band since it is possible for a patient o be wearing the wrong ID band. If there is no ID band, notify the nurse and have her confirm the patient's identity and attach an ID band before the blood is drawn. If there is any discrepancy on the ID band, information given by the patient or on the requisition, a reconciliation of the discrepancy must be made before a collection is taken. More than one patient may have the same name. Usually a name alert is placed on the chart but not in all cases.

Patient identification and consent procedures

The patient identification and consent procedures that are legally required before attempting venipuncture are as follows:
1. If the patient requires an interpreter, get one.
2. Identify yourself to the patient.
3. Tell the patient which doctor requested the blood sample.
4. Explain in general terms what you are going to do.
5. Check the patient's armband or health card to confirm identity.
6. Verify the correct spelling of the patient's name and date of birth.
7. If there is any discrepancy between the patient's written identification and your requisition, STOP. Get a doctor or nurse who knows the patient to confirm the identity, and note this on the requisition.
8. A conscious, adult patient has the right to refuse treatment. If you proceed with collection after the patient has refused it, you can be charged with battery. Mark "PATIENT REFUSED" with your initials, the date and time on the requisition, return

it to the patient's chart, and inform the charge nurse at once. If the patient is unconscious, the law considers you have been given implied consent.

Location of veins

- Great saphenous- runs the entire length of the lower extremity and is the longest vein in the body
- Popliteal- runs deep behind the knee
- Femoral- runs deep in the upper part of the leg
- Lesser saphenous- runs lateral to the ankle, up the leg and deep behind the knee

Choice of vein

First choice would be the median cubital due to its large size, and it usually doesn't bruise severely. Next choice would be the cephalic vein since it does not roll as easily as other veins. A last resort vein would be the basilica vein because it rolls easily and is positioned so that the brachial artery and a major nerve are at risk for puncture if used. Ankle and foot veins should only be punctured at the discretion of a physician and should only be used when no other veins are appropriate. Poor circulation and clotting factors may affect results of tests and cause puncture wounds that may not readily heal.

Recommended sites and methods for retrieving blood

Skin puncture is the preferred method for retrieving blood from a child or infant because children have smaller quantities of blood than adults which can lead to anemia if enough blood is drawn. Also, a child or infant may be hurt if they need to be restrained during a venipuncture. Also, infants may go into cardiac arrest if more than 10% of their blood volume is removed. If a child moves around during venipuncture, it may result in an injury to nerves, veins, and arteries.

NCCLS states that the safest areas for skin puncture in an infant are on the plantar surface of the hell, medial to the imaginary line extending from the middle of the big toe to the heel or lateral to an imaginary line extending from between the fourth and fifth toes to the heel. Deep punctures of an infant's heel can lead to osteochondritis (inflammation of the bone and cartilage) and osteomyelitis (inflammation of the bone).

The recommended site for skin puncture for older children and adults is the fleshy portion on the palmar surface of the distal segment of the middle or ring finger.

Inappropriate sites

The following are some variables that make a site inappropriate for selection:
- Injuries to the skin such as burns, scars, and tattoos
- Damaged veins from repeated collections or drug use
- Swelling (edema)
- Hematoma (Bruising
- Mastectomy or cancer removal including skin cancer

Drawing blood via venipuncture

Position the patient's arm on a pillow so blood flows downwards. Tell the patient to remain still. Retract the skin from the site, so it does not clog the bevel. Uncap the 21 or 22 gauge cannula. Rest the first tube inside the holder. Do not push it onto the hub. Insert the cannula, bevel up, into the vein at a 30° angle. Grasp the holder with one hand. Push the tube onto the hub with the other. Blood flows automatically into the evacuated tube when the stopper is pierced, and stops when its vacuum is depleted. Detach the filled tube from the end of the cannula. Invert the tube several times to mix the anticoagulant and blood. Place the filled tube in the kidney basin. Release the tourniquet to relax the pressure, so blood does not spurt when you remove the cannula from the patient's arm. Rest cotton over the puncture site. Remove the cannula while still on the end of its holder, without unscrewing it. Apply steady pressure to the wound for 4 to 6 minutes to stop bleeding – longer if the patient is taking anticoagulant drugs like aspirin or coumadin. Ask the alert patient to continue applying pressure after the first minute, so you can dispose of the used equipment. Elevate the puncture slightly to help slow bleeding, but do not bend the arm. Apply a band-aid.

Arterial puncture

Common sites
The radial artery is the preferred choice for arterial puncture. It is located on the thumb site of the wrist and is most commonly used. The brachial artery is second choice. It is located in the medial anterior aspect of the antecubital area near the biceps tendon insertion. Femoral artery is only used by physicians and trained ER personnel. It is usually used in emergency situations or with patients with low cardiac output. The ulnar artery is very rarely to never used in arterial puncture. The ulnar artery provides collateral circulation for the hand. Since the radial artery is most commonly used in arterial puncture, the ulnar artery is there as a back up to provide blood to the hand if the radial artery is damaged and becomes unable to supply blood to the hand.

Applying pressure afterward
For 3 to 5 minutes directly after the needle is withdrawn from an arterial puncture, a phlebotomist should apply pressure to the puncture site. A patient should not be allowed to hold pressure since they may not hold adequate pressure for the required length of time.

Faint or no pulse afterward
If you are unable to find a pulse after an arterial puncture or the pulse is faint, blood flow may be blocked partially or completely by a blood clot. Notify the patient's nurse or physician STAT so that circulation can begin to be restored as quickly as possible.

Equipment and assembly for blood collection

Selection of equipment should be done after finding the collection site. This allows you to waste less equipment if your collection site turns out to be inappropriate for the equipment you have assembled. Also, this allows for adequate drying time for the alcohol which allows for proper cleaning of the site and reduced sting from the alcohol. A site should have a minimum drying time of 30 seconds.

Routine adult venipuncture equipment:
- Completed requisition with a physician's signature and billing information
- Soap, water, and towels for hand washing
- Sufficient evacuated blood tubes with the right color stopper
- One 21g or 22g cannula X 1.5" length
- Plastic Vacutainer holder with a luer-lock hub
- Isopropyl alcohol or povidone-iodine swab
- Clean, dry cotton balls
- Band-aid or Micropore tape, if the patient is allergic to adhesive
- Tourniquet (rubber Penrose catheter or blood pressure cuff)
- Kidney basin or tray to hold the specimen during collection
- Latex or vinyl gloves
- Pen with indelible ink
- Plastic biohazard bag with outer pouch for the requisition
- Well-buttoned lab coat to protect your clothing
- Reclining chair or bed to support the patient
- Certain tests require chemical additives, ice, or a hot water bath
- Sharps disposal container
- Garbage can

Gauge of needle and needle selection

The gauge of a needle is a number that is inversely correlates to the diameter of the internal space of the needle for example the larger the needle the smaller the internal space of the needle and the smaller the number the larger the internal space of the needle. Since color-coding varies between manufactures, be careful of using this method to determine the gauge of a needle. When selecting a needle for venipuncture, there are several factors to consider which include the type of procedure, the condition and size of the patient's vein, and the equipment being used. The length of the needle used is determined by the depth of the vein. Keep in mind that the smaller the gauge the larger the bore. The 21-gauge needle is the standard needle used for routine venipuncture.

Colored tube stoppers and additives

The following are the additives that are found with each colored tube stopper:
- Yellow – SPS and ACD
- Red (glass tube) – no additive
- Light blue – sodium citrate
- Lavender – EDTA
- Dark Green – heparin
- Gray – potassium oxalate and sodium fluoride
- Gold –silica, thixotropic gel
- Mottled red and gray - silica, thixotropic gel

Disinfectant and antiseptic

Disinfectants are used to kill possible pathogens. They are bactericidal corrosive compounds composed of chemicals. Some disinfectants are capable of killing viruses such as

HIV and HBV. These are not used on humans to disinfect skin. A common disinfectant is bleach in a 1:10 dilution. Antiseptics are chemical compounds that inhibit or prevent the growth of microorganism microbes usually applied externally. Antiseptics attempt to prevent sepsis but do not necessarily kill bacteria and viruses. Antiseptics are used on human skin. Common antiseptics include70% isopropyl alcohol, betadine, and benzalkonium chloride, with isopropyl alcohol being the most commonly used. Betadine is used when a sterile draw is needed.

Anticoagulant and antiglycolytic additives

The blood collection additives used as anticoagulants and antiglycolytics are as follows:
- Anticoagulant
  - EDTA
  - Citrates
  - Heparin
  - Oxalates
- Antiglycolytic Agent
  - Sodium fluoride
  - Lithium iodoacetate

PPT, SST, and PST

All three tubes contain thixotropic gel which is a non-reactive synthetic substance that serves as an actual physical barrier between the serum and the cellular portion of a specimen after the specimen has been centrifuged. If thixotropic gel is used in tube with EDTA, it is referred to as a plasma preparation tube (PPT.) When thixotropic gel is used in serum collection tube, the gel is referred to as serum separator thus the tube and the gel are called the serum separator tube (SST.) When thixotropic gel is used in a tube with heparin, it is called plasma separator. Thus when thixotropic gel and heparin are in a tube; the tube is called the plasma separator tube (PST.)

Tourniquet

A tourniquet is used to aid in the collection of a blood specimen. The tourniquet is tied in such a way that it is easily removed above the venipuncture site. The purpose of the tourniquet is to slow down venous flow away from the puncture site and to not inhibit arterial flow to the puncture site. By doing this, the vein enlarges to make it easier to locate and puncture. A tourniquet should not be left on longer than 1 minute because this may change the composition of the blood and make testing inaccurate.

Heparin

The anticoagulant heparin works by inhibiting thrombin which is required during the coagulation process. Thrombin is needed to form fibrin from fibrinogen. Thus when thrombin is inhibited a fibrin clot is less likely to develop. The purpose of heparin is to prevent coagulation. The three types of heparin are ammonium, sodium and lithium. Ammonium heparin is used for hematocrit determinations and is found in capillary tubes. Sodium heparin and lithium heparin are used in evacuated tubes. Just be sure that the heparin that is being used is not what is being tested. For example heparin is used for electrolyte testing, but sodium is a commonly tested electrolyte thus sodium heparin would not be an appropriate heparin to use to test for electrolytes. It is important to mix heparin tubes properly to prevent microclots.

Needle safety devices

Needle safety devices protect the needle user's hand by having it remain behind the needle during use and by providing a barrier between the user's hand and the needle after use. Also, the needle safety devices are operable with using a one-handed technique and provide a permanent barrier around the contaminated needle.

Syringe system

Syringe system

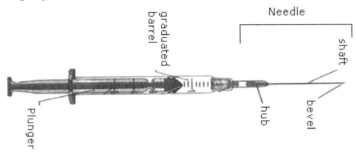

Preparation for venipuncture

The preparation steps for venipuncture are as follows:
1.   Check the expiration dates on all tubes, cannulae and swabs. Get fresh products if any have expired.
2.   Wash, dry, and glove your hands.
3.   Place the equipment in the kidney basin on an easily accessible table, not on the bed where they can break if the patient rolls over.
4.   Select the patient's arm that has no intravenous fluid drip or injury.
5.   Tie the tourniquet around the patient's bicep, or inflate a blood pressure cuff to 20 mm/Hg.
6.   Ask the patient to clench a fist. Palpate the veins in the ante cubital fossa.
7.   If the arm turns blue, or if the patient complains the tourniquet is too tight, loosen it immediately. Wait until the arm returns to a normal color before reapplying. Prolonged or repeated use of the tourniquet or blood pressure cuff can result in artificially high calcium levels in the specimen.

Order of draw

Blood collection tubes must be drawn in a specific order to avoid cross-contamination of additives between tubes. The recommended order of draw is:
- First - blood culture tube (yellow-black stopper)
- Second - non-additive tube (red stopper or SST)
- Third - coagulation tube (light blue stopper). If just a routine coagulation assay is the only test ordered, then a single light blue stopper tube may be drawn. If there is

a concern regarding contamination by tissue fluids or thromboplastins, then one may draw a non-additive tube first, and then the light blue stopper.

- Last draw - additive tubes in this order:
  - SST (red-gray, or gold, stopper). Contains a gel separator and clot activator.
  - Sodium heparin (dark green stopper)
  - PST (light green stopper). Contains lithium heparin anticoagulant and a gel separator.
  - EDTA (lavender stopper)
  - ACDA or ACDB (pale yellow stopper). Contains acid citrate dextrose.
  - Oxalate/fluoride (light gray stopper)

Blood collection by capillary puncture

Capillary puncture is suitable when a very small quantity of blood is required and the patient has difficult veins. Examples of when capillary puncture is appropriate include:

- Newborn PKU
- Diabetic glucose via glucometer
- Anemic hemoglobin via hemoglobinometer
- Bleeding time before surgery

Capillary puncture is inappropriate for blood cultures or large quantities because the site clots quickly. Perform newborn capillary puncture with a short point lancet on the lateral or medial plantar heel surface to avoid nicking the calcaneous (heel bone) and causing osteomyelitis. The infant may require a foot amputation if the site becomes gangrenous. Older infants can have the plantar surface of their big toes pricked with a short point lancet. Children and adults have the distal phalanx palmar surface pricked with a long point lancet.

Wash the puncture site with warm water to dilate capillaries. If the site remains cold, apply a chemical warming pack, such as Hot Shots used by skiers in their gloves. Wrap the pack in a cloth so it does not directly contact the infant's thin skin. Swab the site with alcohol. Puncture the skin quickly with a lancet. Draw blood into the Microtainer tube by capillary action and GENTLE squeezing in this order:

Color	Additive	Order of Draw	# of Inversions
Dark Green	Lithium Heparin	Second	Mix 10 times
Gold and Amber	SST	Fourth	Do not mix
Lavender	EDTA	First	Mix 20 times
Mint Green	PST	Third	Mix 10 times
Red	None	Last	Do not mix

The order of draw is different than that used for venipuncture because capillary blood is more likely to clot or hemolyze during collection. Wiping the puncture with alcohol to encourage bleeding when the wound has already clotted will dilute the specimen. Vigorous squeezing can cause interstitial fluid to leak into the specimen and dilute it, or hemolysis of red blood cells, giving a false result.

Nonblood fluid specimens

Several nonblood fluid specimens are routinely collected for analysis from the human body:
- Urine
- Amniotic Fluid
- Cerebrospinal Fluid
- Gastric Secretions
- Nasopharyngeal Secretions
- Saliva
- Semen
- Serous Fluids
- Sputum
- Sweat
- Synovial Fluid

Urine tests

The following are some common urine tests and what they are commonly used to find:
- Routine Urinalysis
- Culture and Sensitivity – diagnosis urinary tract infection
- Cytology Studies – presence of abnormal cells from urinary tract
- Drug Screening – detects illegal use of drugs (prescription or illicit) and steroid, also monitors therapeutic drug use.
- Pregnancy Test – confirms pregnancy by testing for the presence of HCG

The following aspects of urine are reviewed in a routine urinalysis:
- Physical- color, odor, transparency, specific gravity
- Chemical- looking for bacteria, blood, WBC, protein, and glucose
- Microscopic – urine components i.e. casts, cells, and crystals

<u>24 hour urine specimen collection</u>
All urine must be collected over the course of 24 hours. A large collection container is given to the patient. When a patient awakes, the first void of the morning is for the previous 24 hours and must be discarded. The next void is collected as well as the next void over the next 24 hours as well as the next morning void. Sometimes the specimen collection has to be refrigerated.

<u>Midstream urine collection and midstream clean-catch urine collection</u>
Both involve an initial void into the toilet, interruption of urine flow, the restart of urination into a collection container, collection of a sufficient amount of specimen, and voiding of excess urine down the toilet. The clean-catch involves cleaning of the genital area, collecting urine into a sterile container and quick processing to prevent overgrowth of microorganisms, degradation of the specimen, and incorrect results.

<u>Urine collection from a Foley catheter</u>
When collecting a urine specimen from a catheter bag, care must be taken to ensure germs are not introduced into the Foley tubing as this may cause a urinary tract infection. Wash your hands, don a pair of gloves, and explain to the patient what you are going to do. Clamp the catheter tubing 6 inches above the drainage bag, and allow urine to collect in the tubing.

Thoroughly clean the collection hub with an alcohol swab. Carefully access the collection hub using a Luer-Lok syringe. Collect the desired amount of urine. Transfer the urine from the syringe into the specimen cup, taking care not to touch the cup with the syringe. Tightly close the lid of the specimen cup, and place it in a lab specimen bag. Unclamp the catheter tubing. Dispose of the syringe. Remove the gloves, and wash your hands.

<u>Clean-catch urine specimen</u>
Care must be taken while collecting a urine specimen to make sure that it does not become contaminated during the collection process. A clean-catch urine specimen can be collected from a patient who is able to void. Provide the patient with a sterile specimen cup. Instruct the patient to wash his hands and perineal area thoroughly prior to voiding. The patient should start the stream of urine and urinate for at least 2 seconds before beginning to collect urine in the cup. Don a pair of gloves. Once the patient has acquired a suitable specimen, close the specimen cup tightly and place it in a lab specimen bag. Encourage the patient to wash his hands. Remove the gloves, and wash your hands.

<u>Urinalysis</u>
Below are the common urine dipstick tests in routine urinalysis. Normal values are bracketed:

- Blood (negative): Intact or hemolyzed red blood cells indicate bleeding due to infection, menstruation, paroxysmal hemoglobinuria, or trauma.
- Glucose (negative): Uncontrolled diabetes and women with gestational diabetes spill sugar into their urine when their renal threshold is exceeded.
- Ketones (negative): Uncontrolled diabetes, extreme dieters, and starving people produce ketones in urine when their bodies burn fat instead of sugar.
- Leukocytes (negative): White blood cells indicate bleeding due to infection.
- pH (5 to 9): Acidic urine helps the bladder resist infection. Alkaline urine encourages bacterial growth.
- Protein (up to 8 mg/dl): Albumin is shed from the kidneys if the nephrons are damaged. Trace protein can be from genitals or feces.
- Nitrites (negative): Some bacteria, like E-coli, produce nitrites after eating nitrates, so this is an indicator of infection.

If kidney stones, infection, or damage are suspected, then a microscopic urinalysis is performed with the routine urinalysis (R&M) for casts, crystals, and cells.

Stool collection

A stool specimen is collected from the patient if there is suspicion of an infection or bleeding in the bowels. When the patient needs to move his bowels, wash your hands, don a pair of gloves, and explain to the patient what you are going to do. Position a hat in the commode to catch stool without catching urine as well. Assist the patient to the bedside commode, provide privacy, and allow him to move his bowels. After assisting the patient back to bed, place a small amount of stool into a sterile specimen cup and close the lid tightly. Place the specimen cup into a lab collection bag. Dispose of the remaining stool and the hat. Remove your gloves, and wash your hands.

<u>O&P and pinworm</u>
Stool for ova and parasites (O&P) means the lab looks for worms (helminthes) and protozoa that can cause anemia in feces samples, such as tapeworm and round worms. Give the patient a clean jar containing an ounce of formalin. Tell the patient to use a popsicle stick to mix a teaspoon of stool with the preservative and return it, tightly capped and labeled, to the lab.

Pinworms are white, thread-like parasites usually contracted by children from sand boxes in which infected cats and dogs have defecated. The child often scratches his/her itchy bottom and grinds the teeth while sleeping. Give the parent a stool container containing a pinworm paddle, or tell the parent to use a jar with clear tape. When the child sleeps, use a flashlight to visualize the anus. Female tapeworms leave the bowel to lay eggs around the anus at night. Gently touch the paddle or tape to the anus and place it in the jar. Cap tightly. Wash hands well. Return the labeled jar to the lab.

<u>Occult blood and guaiac</u>
Patients who use Aspirin regularly or have ulcers may lose microscopic amounts of blood in their feces. The lab examines stool smears on a mail-in card for occult blood. Give your patient an occult blood kit. Tell him or her to follow the enclosed diet for three days before collection, as foods that cause bleeding must be avoided (e.g., cantaloupe, turnip, broccoli and horseradish). Tell the patient to place plastic wrap under the toilet seat and defecate. Use the enclosed popsicle sticks to smear thin samples of stool from three consecutive bowel movements on the three windows in the card. The patient mails the card back to the lab in the envelope provided.

Guaiac also detects occult blood, but is collected by the doctor in the office during a rectal examination with a gloved finger. The doctor wipes the soiled glove across a window that contains guaiac resin on a card and adds two drops of peroxide. If the sample oxidizes (turns blue) in 2 seconds or less, the patient is losing blood. These two tests are not reliable for bowel cancer.

Sputum culture

Sputum is phlegm (mucous) and other matter expelled from the lungs and trachea. It should contain as little saliva from the mouth as possible. Sputum can be cultured (C&S) to identify an infection, such as pneumonia. Sputum can be examined microscopically to identify cancer or a disease-causing agent, such as asbestos fibers. If the doctor orders sputum for AFB (acid fast bacilli stain), then the lab searches for bacteria that cause tuberculosis. Drink fluids the night before specimen collection, to encourage secretions. Collect the specimen upon arising, because sputum collects in the air passageways during sleep. Tap on the chest. Cough deeply. If you cannot produce any sputum, try inhaling steaming salt water. If any sputum arises, spit it into a sterile cup. Cap it tightly and label it. Bring the sputum to the lab immediately for testing. If you cannot transport it immediately, refrigerate it up to 3 days. Sometimes the doctor orders specimen collection on 3 consecutive days. The patient should be instructed to drink fluids the night before specimen collection to encourage secretions. The specimen should be collected upon arising because sputum collects in the air passageway during sleep. The chest should be tapped and the patient should be instructed to cough deeply. If sputum is not produced, the patient should be instructed to try inhaling steaming salt water. If any sputum arises, the patient should be instructed to spit it into a sterile cup. The cup should be capped tightly and labeled.

C&S

Sensitivity testing is also called culture and susceptibility testing (C&S). Wash your hands. Don gloves and a lab coat. Sterilize a loop. Streak body fluid (stool, urine, blood, sputum, or wound drainage) across an agar plate with the loop. Rotate the loop and streak again so the bacteria are evenly distributed across the agar. You may also place tissue on media. Incubate at body temperature (37°C) for 24 to 48 hours. If growth occurs, the lab distinguishes normal flora from pathogens by chemical and enzyme tests. A lab tech inoculates pathogens with antimicrobials to see if they can be killed (susceptible), or cannot be killed (resistant). If the antimicrobial that works best requires high doses (intermediate), it is likely to be toxic to the patient. The doctor initially prescribes the antimicrobial to which the pathogen is susceptible, except if the patient is allergic to it. The doctor consults with a pharmacist and microbiologist to choose the least toxic alternative, but the intermediate dose may need to be given over a long time and the patient may suffer side-effects. If the pathogen is resistant to many antimicrobials, then expensive intravenous combination therapy may be the only effective treatment.

Manual hemoglobin test for a hemodialysis patient

Test the hemoglobinometer with known controls first. Polish a clean hemocytometer slide with lens paper. Fill a blue-ringed, unheparinized capillary tube with blood. Place one drop of blood on the hemocytometer slide. Roll the heparinized, wooden hemolysis stick over the blood drop until the blood is hemolyzed and transparent (about 30 seconds). Place the cover slip over the slide. Slide them together into the hemoglobinometer. Look through the viewer. Adjust the light until the two fields you see are exactly the same color. (Most hemoglobinometers use green and black.) Read the scale (usually on the side of the meter) and record the hemoglobin level. (Normal values are 12—16 g/dl for women, and 14—16 g/dl for men.) Disassemble the slide and cover slip. Sanitize, disinfect, polish, and case them. Wipe the test area and outside of the hemoglobinometer with disinfectant. Hemoglobinometer readings with capillary blood show about 10% false-positives for anemia, as compared to venous Coulter Counter readings. Hemoglobinometers are for point-of-care testing for "ballpark" estimates.

Hematocrit test

A hematocrit (Hct) test separates the blood cells from the plasma in a centrifuge as part of a complete blood count (CBC). Hct indirectly measures red blood cell (RBC) mass, so if the RBCs are of normal size, then the Hct should confirm the RBC count. Patients with macrocytic, microcytic, or iron deficiency anemia with small RBCs will not have parallel Hct and RBC counts. Report results as Packed Cell Volume (PCV), meaning the percentage by volume of packed red blood cells in whole blood. Normal values for venous blood are: Males 42% to 52%; females 36% to 48%. Microhematocrit readings from capillary tubes are a little higher. Babies have higher hematocrits than adults because they have more macrocytic RBC's. An abnormal hematocrit suggests follow-up tests must be done for a firm diagnosis. Low hematocrit readings (less than 30%) may indicate many diseases: Adrenal insufficiency, anemia, burns, Hodgkin's disease, leukemia, or poisoning. High hematocrit can be from erythrocytosis, polycythemia vera, or shock.

Glucose tolerance test

Preparation
A patient should eat balanced meals with 150 grams of carbohydrates for 3 days and should refrain from eating 12 hours before the test as well as not smoking or chewing gum before or during the testing period.

Arterial blood pH

7.35-7.45 is the normal range for arterial blood pH. Acidosis describes below normal blood pH. Alkalosis describes above normal blood pH. pH is the measure of the acidity of a solution. pH is equal to the negative logarithm of the concentration of hydrogen ions in a solution. A pH of 7 is neutral. Values less than 7 are acidic, and values greater than 7 are basic. A range of 6.5 to 7.5 is considered a neutral environment.

Allen test

The purpose of the Allen's test is to determine the presence of collateral circulation in the hand by the ulnar artery.
    1. Compress the radial and ulnar arteries with fingers while the patient makes a fist.
    2. Patient opens hand; it should have a blanched appearance.
    3. The ulnar artery is released and the patient's hand should flush with color. If this occurs, the patient has a positive Allen test and has collateral circulation of the ulnar artery.

Electrolyte analysis

Bicarbonate, chloride, potassium and sodium are the four most commonly tested for electrolytes.

Centers for Disease Control guidelines for correct specimen processing

When the PCT encounters a doctor's order to collect, ship, or store an unfamiliar specimen or vaccine, then he/she should visit the Web site for the Centers for Disease Control at http://emergency.cdc.gov/labissues/#shipping. Scroll through the alphabetical lists of infectious agents and chemical terrorism agents. The CDC's charts briefly explain how to safely collect, store, plate, stain and transport dangerous biological materials. Often, the CDC also estimates the patient's chance of recovery. Your employer may decide to use dangerous biological agents and toxins for research. If these materials are a serious threat to human, animal or plant life, then you must register them with the National Select Agent Registry. Obtain the necessary registration forms and advice at http://www.selectagents.gov/index.html

Prognosis and test details

The patient care technician's responsibility is not to inform a patient of his prognosis; this is the responsibility of the patient's physician. The patient care technician may not know all the facts of the case and may give false and detrimental information to the patient. Encourage the patient to ask the physician about the prognosis. When asked about a collection being drawn, do not discuss in detail what is being tested for since there can be various reasons why a test was ordered by the patient's physician. Respond to the patient that the physician has ordered these test as a part of the patient's medical care and that if they have any questions about them please ask the physician.

Drawing blood from a sleeping patient

Drawing blood from a sleeping patient is inappropriate. It may startle the patient and may change testing results. Also, you or the patient could be injured as the result of the patient being startled. The appropriate action to take would be to gently say the patient's name and shake the bed (never the patient) to wake them up.

Basal state

The basal state is defined at the condition of the body early in the morning while the body is at rest and has been fasting for about 12 hours. For example, a patient who ate dinner at 5:00PM and wakes at 5:00AM is close to his or her body's basal state. The factors that may influence basal state are age, altitude, daily variations, dehydration, diet, drugs (prescription and illegal), exercise, fever, gender, humidity, jaundice, position, pregnancy, smoking, stress, and temperature.

Issues affecting blood collection

Many patients have allergies. These include possible allergies to adhesives, latex, and antiseptics. A patient may have a bleeding or bruising disorder that results from a genetic reason or medication that they are taking. Some patients may faint (syncope) during a procedure. It is very appropriate to recline a patient or have the lay down if they have fainted before. Some patients have a fear of needles. Some may experience nausea and vomiting from fear or an illness they have. It may be necessarily to have a trash can or spit-up container nearby for easy access. If a patient his overweight or obese then it may make a collection difficult.

Risks from blood collections complications or errors

The following are some of the risks to patients if a complication or error results from blood collection:
- Arterial puncture
- Anemia resulting from the procedure
- Infection
- Hematoma (bruising) of the venipuncture site
- Damage to a nerve if punctured
- Vein damage
- Pain

Hematoma
Hematoma can result from errors in phlebotomy techniques:
- inadequate pressure to the collection site after a blood draw
- blood leaking through the back of a vein that was pierced
- blood leaking from a partial pierced vein
- an artery is pierced

Wiping away the first droplet of blood

The first droplet of blood contains excess tissue fluid which may affect test results. Also, the alcohol residue on the skin will be wiped away with the first droplet of blood. The alcohol can hemolyze the blood specimen and keep a round droplet of blood from forming.

Acceptable blood smear

A blood smear will be spread over one-half to three-fourths of the slide. There will be a gradual shift from thick to thin blood smear on the slide with the thinnest part of the slide being one blood cell thick. This thinnest part of the blood smear is sometimes referred to as the "feather." The feather part of the blood smear is the most important since the differential is performed there. In blood smears made using the two slide method hold the slide that will smear the blood droplet at a 30 degree angle to the slide that the blood droplet was placed on.

LIS

An LIS is a laboratory information system. Usually the LIS is used to order tests, print labels for specimens, and enter test results. LIS can be customized to specific laboratory requirements.

Information on a computer-generated label

The label would contain the patient's name, date of birth or age, medical record number, collection time (in military time).

Inverting a tube

A tube should be inverted if it contains an additive and if the manufacturer's instructions require for it to be inverted. If the tube is a nonadditive tube then it does not have to be inverted. An additive tube usually is inverted between three and eight times to properly mix the additive with the blood.

Chilling specimens

The most appropriate way to chill a specimen is to immerse it into an ice and water slush. Ice cubes alone will not allow for adequate cooling of the specimen, and where the ice cubes touch the specimen may freeze it resulting in possible hemolysis or breakdown of the analyte.

Importance of proper handling of specimens

46 to 68% of lab errors result from improper handling of a specimen before it was analyzed. For example, if an anticoagulant tube is improperly mixed, it may result in microclots forming. If a tube is shaken too hard hemolysis of the specimen may occur. If a specimen is not cooled properly then metabolic processes may continue after collection which may skew test results.

Aliquot

When a specimen is collected, it may need to be divided to run several test on it. An aliquot is a fraction of the specimen. Each aliquot has its own tube for testing and is label with the same information as the original specimen.

Rejection of specimens

Some reasons why a specimen may be rejected for testing include incorrect or incomplete identification, collected in an expired tube, inadequate amount of specimen collected (QNS, quantity not sufficient), and collection in an incorrect tube.

Putting on sterile gloves

Sterile gloves must be put on carefully to ensure germs are not introduced onto the sterile surface. Wash your hands, and dry them thoroughly. Unfold the package of gloves, and lay it on a flat surface. Using your nondominant hand, grasp the glove intended for your dominant hand at the fold of the cuff. Cup the fingers of your dominant hand, and carefully slide it into the glove. If the glove needs adjustments, wait until both gloves are on before making them. Using your dominant hand in the sterile glove, slide your fingers beneath the cuff of the remaining glove. Carefully slide the fingers of your nondominant hand into the glove. Make any necessary adjustments. Do not touch any non-sterile surfaces, and keep your hands above your waist to maintain sterility.

Important terms

- Accession Number - Unique number given for each test request
- Aerosol - Substance released in the form of a fine mist
- Barcode - Series of black bars and white spaces spaced at intentional, unique distances to represent numbers and letters
- Bevel - Slanted tip of a needle used to puncture the skin and vein without removing a piece of the vein.
- Blood smear - Blood layer on a glass slide made from a drop of blood
- Capillary blood gases - Blood gases retrieved from an arterialized skin puncture
- Centrifugation - The process of substance separation by spinning
- Hub - End of a needle that attaches to the blood collection device i.e. syringe or tube holder
- Impermeable - Does not allow the passage of liquids
- Interstitial fluid - Liquid found between cells
- Intracellular fluid - Liquid found within cell membranes
- Plunger - The part of the syringe that when pulled on creates a vacuum allowing the barrel of the syringe to be filled with fluid or air.
- Shaft - The hollow round long cylinder-shaped part of a needle
- Sharps container - An easily sealed, rigid, leak-proof, puncture-resistant, disposable box with a locking lid in which used needles and sharp materials are disposed.

Patient Care Responsibilities

Vital signs

Stable vital signs in the normal range indicate good health (homeostasis). Ill or injured patients have vital signs outside the normal range. The severity of the illness or injury often is indicated by the variability of vital sign measurements. Look for variations from previous visits. Wide variations mean the patient is unstable; check the vital signs every 5 minutes. In stable patients, check the vital signs every 15 minutes.

The five vital signs that are most commonly measured are temperature, pulse, respiration rate, blood pressure, and pain level. Temperature measures the patient's core body temperature. Pulse measures the number of times the patient's heart beats per minute. Respiration rate measures the number of times the patient breathes every minute. Blood pressure is recorded as two numbers. The top number is referred to as the systolic pressure; it measures the pressure within the patient's arteries during contraction of the heart. The bottom number is the diastolic blood pressure; this number reflects the pressure within the arteries while the heart is at rest between each contraction. Pain level measures the presence or absence of pain. It indicates the severity of that pain according to the patient.

Pulse

The pulse is a surge of blood through an artery that occurs when the heart contracts (systole).

Pulse rate varies by age:

Normal Resting Pulse Rate	Age
60—100 beats per minute	Adult
80—100 beats per minute	Child
100 beats per minute	Toddler
100—140 beats per minute	Infant under one year
up to 150 beats per minute	Newborn (neonate)

The key pulse points are:
1. Apical over the heart
2. Brachial in the elbow bend (for children under 1 year)
3. Carotid in the neck (for unconscious patients)
4. Dorsalis pedis on top of the foot
5. Facial on the jaw under the mouth
6. Femoral in the thigh
7. Popliteal on the back of the knee
8. Posterior tibial on the back of the ankle
9. Radial on the wrist below the thumb (most common in patients older than 1 year)
10. Temporal on the temple
11. Ulnar on the wrist below the little finger

Use direct pressure on the pulse point nearest a cut to control bleeding. Evaluate the extremities for healthy circulation by palpating the distal pulses. The doctor rubs the carotid arteries on both sides of the patient's neck as vagus nerve stimulation (VNS) therapy to decrease pulse rate in tachycardia.

If you cannot feel a distal pulse in your patient's limbs, find the apical pulse in the chest. Count to the 5th rib space in the middle of the left side of the chest or midclavicular line. If the apical pulse is *regular*, count for 30 seconds and record the reading. If the apical pulse is *irregular*, count for a full minute and record the reading. Report an irregular pulse to the doctor to evaluate for possible pulse deficit. A pulse deficit occurs when the radial pulse in the wrist is slower than the apical pulse in the chest. A pulse deficit can indicate your patient has weak heart contractions, which fail to transmit beats to the arterial system.

Peripheral pulse
Wash your hands, greet the patient, and explain what you are going to do. Check the patient's identity using his armband. Take the patient's hand, and slide your index and middle finger along the thumb, up to the hollow of the wrist. Apply gentle pressure until you can feel the pulse. If the patient's heart rate is regular, count the number of beats for 30 seconds and multiply that number by two. If the patient's heart rate is irregular, count the number of beats for a full minute. Record the number in the patient's chart. Wash your hands.

Apical pulse
An apical pulse measures the number of times the heart beats every minute by auscultating at the apex of the heart. Wash your hands, greet the patient, and explain what you are going to do. Verify the patient's identity using his armband. Place the bell of the stethoscope against the patient's left chest and locate the area in which the pulse is the loudest. If the patient's heart rate is regular, count the number of beats for 30 seconds and multiply by two. If the patient's heart rate is irregular, count the number of beats for a full minute. Record the patient's pulse, clean the stethoscope, and wash your hands.

Indications of an abnormal pulse
The normal pulse range for an adult is between 60 and 80 beats per minute. The patient may have a low heart rate if he is physically fit or if he is resting. Some medications may also decrease the patient's heart rate. An elevated heart rate may be the result of exercise, stress, drugs, or caffeine. Certain medications may also elevate the patient's heart rate. If the patient has an elevated temperature or an infection, the heart rate will be elevated. An elevated heart rate can also be the result of uncontrolled bleeding.

Tachycardia and bradycardia

Tachycardia is a pulse rate over 100 beats per minute, which may be caused by: Anxiety; fear; stress; pneumonia; anemia; low blood pressure; dehydration; hyperthyroidism; and heart conditions. Bradycardia is a resting heart rate less than 60 beats per minute, which may be caused by: Heart attack (MI); hypothermia; heat exhaustion; obstructive jaundice; skull fracture; malnutrition; hypothyroidism; and many adverse drug reactions. Olympic athletes may have bradycardia because their hearts are extremely efficient.

Temperature

A live patient's body temperature is measured to determine if he/she is storing and releasing heat properly, to detect abnormally high or low body temperatures, and to assess the effectiveness of some types of medications. The coroner measures temperature to determine time of death. Human temperature ranges are:
- Ideal 98.6°F (37°C)
- Normal Range 97.8°F (36.5°C) — 99°F (37.2°C)
- Hypothermia (too cold) <95°F (<35°C)
- Pyrexia (fever) >98.6°F oral or >99.8°F rectal
- Hyperpyrexia (lethal fever) 107.6°F (>42°C)

Temperature is lowest around 4:00 a.m. and highest around 6:00 p.m. Temperature spikes occur after meals. Ovulation in women creates a temperature rise of 0.5°F—1°F when measured before arising from bed in the morning (basal body temperature). Individual temperature differences in healthy people are due to the rate of metabolism. Patients with hypothyroidism tend to be cold. Body temperature differs at different sites. Normal oral temperature is 98.6 °F, while normal rectal temperature is 99.6 °F (37.6°C). The mouth is open to the air, so its temperature is lower. Do not take the patient's oral temperature for 30 minutes after eating or drinking, as it will be raised with hot food, and decreased with cold drinks.

Axillary temperature
Wash your hands, don a pair of gloves, and greet the patient. Explain what you are going to do, and verify the patient's identity by checking his armband. Make sure that the area under the patient's arm is dry. Place a plastic sheath over the temperature probe. Position the thermometer in the axillary area, and instruct the patient to keep his arm down. Leave the thermometer in place until it indicates a reading. If a mercury thermometer is being used, allow the thermometer to remain in place for 10 minutes. Record the temperature, remove the gloves, wash your hands, and clean the thermometer prior to using it on another patient.

Oral temperature
Wash your hands, don a pair of gloves, and greet the patient. Explain what you are going to do, and check the patient's armband. Ensure that the patient has not had anything to drink in the past 15 minutes as this will make his temperature read falsely low. Cover the thermometer with a plastic sheath, and place it under the patient's tongue. Instruct the patient to keep his mouth closed and not to talk while the thermometer is obtaining a reading. Wait until the thermometer indicates the temperature has been read. Note the temperature, clean the thermometer, remove your gloves, and wash your hands.

Abnormal temperature
A person's core body temperature is closely regulated to ensure an optimum environment for the complex chemical reactions within the body. The normal temperature range for an adult patient is between 97.8 and 99.1 degrees Fahrenheit. A low core body temperature may indicate the onset of an infection. The patient's temperature may also be low after coming from a cold environment, such as the operating room. The primary cause for an elevated temperature is infection. Because a fever is the result of the immune system mounting a defense against an infection, it may not be necessary to treat the fever unless the temperature goes above 101.5 degrees Fahrenheit.

Rectal temperature

Wash your hands, don a pair of gloves, greet the patient, and explain what you are going to do. Identify the patient using his armband. Place a plastic cover over the temperature probe. Assist the patient into a side lying position. Apply lubrication to the thermometer, and slide it 1 inch into the patient's rectum. Leave it in place until a temperature reads. If you are using a mercury thermometer, leave it in place for 3 minutes. Remove the thermometer, and inspect it to make sure it is still intact. Record the temperature. Position the patient for comfort. Clean the thermometer, remove the gloves, and wash your hands.

Blood pressure

Wash your hands, greet the patient, and explain what you are going to do. Verify the patient's identity using his armband. Wrap the blood pressure cuff around the patient's upper arm, and place the bell of the stethoscope over the brachial artery. Pump the bulb of the blood pressure cuff, inflating the cuff between 150 and 180 mmHg. Slowly release the pressure, while listening through the stethoscope. Note the pressure at which you first hear a pulse; this is the systolic blood pressure. Continue to listen to the pulse. Note the pressure at which the pulse fades away; this is the patient's diastolic blood pressure. Record the findings on the patient's chart, and wash your hands.

Indications of abnormal blood pressure

The normal range for a systolic blood pressure is 110 to 140. The normal range for a diastolic blood pressure is 60 to 90. Hypotension is defined as a systolic blood pressure less than 100 mmHg. The patient may have a low blood pressure because he is resting or as a result of certain medications. Bleeding, infection, heart failure, or dehydration may also result in hypotension. Hypertension is defined as a systolic blood pressure greater than 150 mmHg. The patient may have hypertension as a result of chronic illness, pain, or stress. Hypertension may also be caused by kidney failure, heart disease, or certain neurological disorders.

Orthostatic blood pressure

Orthostatic hypotension is a condition in which the patient's blood pressure drops as a result of a change in position. This can cause dizziness or lightheadedness after standing, which may lead to falls. To check for orthostatic hypotension, measure the patient's blood pressure while he is lying down. Assist the patient into a sitting position, and measure the blood pressure again. If the patient is able to stand, assist him into a standing position and measure the blood pressure a third time. If the patient's blood pressure drops by more than 20 mmHg systolic or 10 mmHg diastolic, then he is considered to have orthostatic hypotension. The nurse should be notified immediately.

Aneroid sphygmomanometer

Blood pressure is measured as systolic and diastolic pressure by means of a stethoscope and an aneroid sphygmomanometer (portable blood pressure cuff). For example, if the reading is 120/80 mm/Hg, 120 is the systole, and 80 is the diastole. The first Korotkoff sound the PCT hears is the systole; the last Korotkoff sound is the diastole. Position the blood pressure cuff so that it surrounds 75% of the patient's upper arm. The width of the cuff bladder should exceed the diameter of the patient's arm by 20% or more. This is about 40% of the circumference of the arm. Fit the cuff so that the bottom edge sits about one inch above the elbow joint. Place the stethoscope's diaphragm over the patient's radial artery, and insert the earpieces into your ears. Inflate the cuff quickly, in 7 seconds or less. Deflate the blood pressure cuff slowly, at a rate of 2—3 mm/Hg per second. Remove the cuff and stethoscope. Record the measurement in your patient's chart immediately.

Values for normal blood pressure, hypertension, and hypotension

Increased blood pressure contributes to stroke and heart disease. Low blood pressure is associated with shock, trauma, bleeding, or severe infection.
- Upper normal adult blood pressure: 120/80 mm/Hg (millimeters of mercury)
- Prehypertension: Systole between 120 and 139 and diastole between 80 and 90
- Borderline hypertension (high blood pressure): 140/90 mm/Hg
- Hypertension Stage 1: Systole between 140 and 159 and diastole between 90 and 99
- Hypertension Stage 2: Systole 160 or more and diastole of 100 or more
- Hypotension (low blood pressure): 90/50 mm/Hg or less

Equipment or technique problems that produce false BP results

False BP results can occur from:
- Incorrect cuff size — If your patient is obese, use a thigh cuff on the upper arm. If your patient is a child, use a pediatric cuff.
- Deflating the cuff more rapidly than 2—3 mm/Hg per second
- Venous congestion makes it difficult to hear the blood pressure sounds. Elevating the patient's arm after positioning the cuff but before inflating it can decrease venous congestion.
- Loud environmental noises
- Operator error

Measuring respirations

Measuring respirations is done to assess the number of times per minute the patient breathes. Typically, when a person is made aware of his breathing, he does not breathe deeply or regularly. Do not tell the patient you are measuring the respiration rate, as it will make him aware of his breathing and may produce an inaccurate result. The ideal time to measure the patient's respiration rate is after checking the patient's pulse. Count the number of times the patient breathes, counting one rise and fall of the chest wall as one respiration. Count the number of breaths for one minute, noting the depth of the breath and any use of accessory muscles. Record the respiratory rate on the patient's chart. Wash your hands.

Indications of abnormal respirations
The normal range for respiration rate is between 12 to 18 breaths per minute. A number of factors may affect the rate of the patient's breathing. The patient may breathe more slowly if he is resting or if he is positioned on his back. Certain narcotics may also depress the respiratory drive, resulting in fewer breaths per minute. A rapid respiration rate may be caused by increased activity, pain, or stress. An elevated temperature or an infection may cause the patient's respiratory rate to be quicker. Other conditions, such as respiratory distress, fluid overload, or a heart attack, may also cause an elevated respiratory rate.

Pulse oximetry

Pulse oximetry non-invasively measures a patient's oxyhemoglobin level during stress tests or emergency medicine, which is much easier for the patient than having painful arterial blood gases (SaO_2) drawn at intervals. Use a pulse oximeter to monitor your at-risk patient's oxygen saturation level (SpO_2) continuously. Attach the oximeter sensor to one of the patient's first three fingers (index, middle or ring). If the patient's hands are damaged, use a toe or earlobe. Consider using the forehead, nose, or other parts of the foot only as a last resort. It should always read between 95% and 100%. An alarm sounds if the SpO_2 falls under 90% -- tell the doctor the patient is hypoxic. Many oximeters also give the patient's heart rate at the same time. A pulse oximeter is not accurate if the patient is very anemic, has poor circulation, is edematous, moves a lot, or wears artificial nails or very dark nail polish. Adjust the room temperature, lighting, and move electronic equipment to get a good reading.

Height and weight

Upright scale
An upright scale can be used to measure the patient's height and weight if he has the strength to stand on the scale. Wash your hands, greet the patient, and explain what you are going to do. Confirm the patient's identity using his armband. Assist the patient to a standing position, and show him to the upright scale. Instruct the patient to stand on the scale, facing away from the scale. Lower the height rod until it rests on top of the patient's head. Make a note of the height. Assist the patient in turning until he is facing the scale. Move the weights on the scale until the bar is balanced; make a note of the patient's weight. Assist the patient back to the chair or bed, and position him for comfort. Wash your hands.

Lying down
A patient who is bed bound will need to have his height and weight measured while in bed. Wash your hands, greet the patient, and explain what you are going to do. Verify the patient's identity using his armband. Obtain assistance from a colleague. Roll the patient onto a bath blanket and the bed scale pad. Prior to obtaining the weight, mark the placement of the patient's heels and the top of his head on the bath blanket. Weigh the patient using the bed scale, and make a note of the patient's weight. Remove the bed scale pad and the bath blanket. Measure the distance between the two marks on the pad, and record that as the patient's height. Reposition the patient for comfort, and wash your hands.

Therapeutic communication

Therapeutic communication is a method of communicating with patients that encourages them to open up and provide information. Because of the level of stress involved in hospitalization, the patient often needs to communicate but is unsure how to initiate conversation with the health care staff. Therapeutic communication combines a variety of verbal and nonverbal communication techniques in order to encourage the patient to speak openly. By making note of the patient's body language as well as his words, the patient care technician can interpret the patient's emotional state and communicate with the patient effectively.

Non-therapeutic communication

Seven examples of non-therapeutic communication are:
1. Negative judgments: "You should stop arguing with the nurses."
2. Devaluing patient's feelings: "Everyone gets upset at times."
3. Disagreeing directly: "That can't be true," or "I think you are wrong."
4. Defending against criticism: "The doctor is not being rude; he's just very busy today."
5. Subject change to avoid dealing with uncomfortable topics:
   Patient: "I'm never going to get well."
   PCT: "Your parents will be here in just a few minutes."
6. Inappropriate literal responses, even as a joke, especially if the patient is at all confused or having difficulty expressing ideas:
   Patient: "There are bugs crawling under my skin."
   PCT: "I'll get some bug spray."
7. Challenge to establish reality, which often just increases confusion and frustration: "If you were dying, you wouldn't be able to yell and kick!"

Verbal communication

Verbal communication is one way in which people communicate. It encompasses what is said as well as the way it is said. When communicating with the patient, the patient care technician should take into account the patient's language and word choice, as well as the tone of voice and the volume at which the words are spoken. When talking with a patient, it is important to think carefully about what you say before you say it as words can often be misunderstood. It is also important to ensure that your comments are appropriate to the setting and conversation.

Nonverbal communication

Any type of message transmitted between two people that does not involve words is non-verbal communication. 85% to 93% of successful communication depends on nonverbal cues. Remember that your patient is likely apprehensive and English may not be his /her first language. Your patient may have difficulty speaking due to injury, drugs, age, deformity, developmental disability, or the instruments used during a procedure. Watch your patient's facial expressions, gestures, posture, and position. Tight posture and/or crossed arms and legs suggest resistance. Conversely, relaxed posture and uncrossed appendages suggest openness. Your posture affects your patient. Sit closely beside your patient, rather than towering directly over him/her in an intimidating manner. Explain what you are going to do. A patient feels more comfortable when he/she is well informed beforehand and the PCT works from the side. Maintain the proper social distance (territoriality) between yourself and your patient during discussions (about 3 feet apart). A patient care technician should closely monitor her own body language to make sure that it does not contradict what she is saying. For example, a patient care technician who talks to the patient while frequently checking her watch is indicating that she is in a hurry. Such body language discourages open communication and should be avoided.

Inappropriate communication techniques

10 inappropriate communications techniques to avoid in therapeutic relationships are as follows:
1. Ask leading questions — Never shape the patient's answers to questions, or try to change the patient's interpretation of the situation by "putting words into the patient's mouth"
2. Demand an explanation — Do not ask "why" questions in an accusing tone
3. Give advice — The physician advises and the PCT supports
4. Demand an immediate response — Allow the patient sufficient time for silent reflection before responding
5. Disinterested body language — Do not appear distracted or make the patient feel inconsequential by impatient motions, bored posture, or rolling your eyes
6. Minimize the patient's feelings — Do not compare feelings and experiences
7. Negatively empower — Do not help your patient to manipulate another person
8. Make false promises — Never promise the patient that the doctor will definitely cure the condition, or make promises that cannot be kept
9. Play into stereotypes — Racist, sexist, and religious prejudice must not influence your treatment of the patient
10. Deliberately mislead — Always disclose upcoming treatments, tests, or procedures

Appropriate communication techniques

4 *appropriate* communication techniques to encourage in therapeutic relationships are as follows:
1. Use active listening — Paraphrase and repeat back information transmitted by your patient. Ask for clarification when the message is confusing. Summarize what you agreed to at the end of your conversation.
2. Watch for nonverbal cues — Nonverbal cues are gestures, grimaces, posturing, appearance, and eye movements that comprise 85% of all communication. Nonverbal cues denote pain, fear, lying, depression, or subterfuge by a caregiver. Gently ask your patient to clarify when verbal and nonverbal cues do not match. Children and psychiatric patients may develop tic disorders (involuntary gestures and movements). If you cannot decipher which movements are truly cues and which are tics, ask the doctor.
3. Ask open-ended questions — Get your patient to 'open up', rather than ask questions that require only a yes or no answer.
4. Consider influences — Put communication in the context of your patient's: Developmental age; emotions; values; ethics; health; education; culture; environment; social and family status; and drug levels.

Components of communication

There are five components that must be present in order for communication to take place. The first component is the sender. The sender is the original source of the message. The next component is the message itself or what the sender is trying to convey. Another component of communication is the channel or the means through which the message is being conveyed. This is typically done using either verbal or nonverbal communication. The fourth component is the receiver or the person who is receiving the message. The final component is feedback or the response to the original message. The role of the sender and the receiver may interchange during the course of a conversation.

Steps to encourage communication

There are a number of steps the patient care technician can take in order to encourage communication with the patient. First, the patient care technician can ensure the patient is in an environment in which he can communicate freely. If the patient is comfortable, he is more likely to participate in therapeutic conversation. The patient care technician should also ensure the patient's privacy during the conversation. The patient may feel embarrassed about sharing personal information in a public setting. The patient care technician should make an effort to appear unhurried, encouraging the patient to talk by sitting near the patient during the conversation. The patient care technician should also convey interest by facing the patient and maintaining eye contact during the conversation.

Silence

Silence can be an effective communication tool because it can convey a number of emotions. While communicating with the patient, silence can convey the sentiment of affection. This type of silence is typically accompanied by nonverbal actions, such as a hug or holding the patient's hand. Silence can also be utilized to encourage the patient to give more information. If this is done during a conversation, the patient may continue to talk to fill the silence. Silence can also give the patient time for contemplation. Care must be taken in utilizing silence as a communication tool as it can sometimes be misinterpreted as hostility or rudeness.

Effective communication

When the patient care technician is talking to the patient, there are a number of ways she can make sure that what she is saying is clearly communicated. The patient care technician should avoid using medical terminology while talking to the patient as many find it to be confusing. The patient care technician should make an effort to use words that can be understood by the layman. For example, instead of saying 'hypertension', the patient care technician can be better understood by using the phrase 'high blood pressure'. If a medical term must be used, the patient care technician should define the term for the patient. While talking with the patient, the patient care technician should speak slowly and clearly in a moderate tone of voice.

Asking questions

Asking questions can be effective in encouraging communication with the patient. There are two types of questions, open-ended and closed-ended. Open-ended questions encourage the patient to provide added detail about the subject of the conversation, while giving him more control over the conversation. "How do you feel about that?" is an example of an open-ended question. Closed-ended questions can be used to focus the conversation or get it back on track. They are typically used to elicit a short answer. An example of a closed-ended question is "What would you like for lunch?"

Active listening

Active listening is the method of listening attentively to the conversation at hand. During a typical conversation, it is not uncommon for a person to not devote her full attention to what is being said. She may be thinking of other things or focusing on the work she is trying to do. When a person is listening actively, she is not only paying attention to the conversation, but also considering the patient's words and forming an appropriate response that will encourage further conversation. Active listening also takes into account various aspects of nonverbal communication in order to draw the appropriate conclusions from the conversation.

Reflecting

Reflecting is another method of encouraging the patient to talk about a particular subject. A patient care technician reflects a statement by repeating all or part of the patient's original statement back to the patient. For example, the patient says, "I feel so lonely." An appropriate reflective response would be "Lonely?" Another form of reflecting is to make a statement regarding the patient's feelings. For example, the patient care technician may say, "It seems like you are very happy about this." This reflects the patient's emotional state and encourages him to speak openly about what he is thinking and feeling.

Restating and using general leads

A general lead is a device used to encourage the patient to continue speaking about a particular subject. Examples of general leads include phrases such as 'go on' or 'I see.' These are effective because they allow the patient to guide the conversation, giving him the opportunity to voice his thoughts and concerns. General leads also indicate that the patient care technician is paying attention to what is being said. When a patient care technician restates something, she rephrases a comment that the patient made earlier in the conversation in order to encourage the patient to elaborate on it. For example, the patient care technician might say, "So you think you have too much equipment on you?" if the patient makes a comment about all of the tubes and wires attached to him.

Communication with disabled patients

The U.S. Department of Labor suggests:
- Gain the person's attention before speaking by gently tapping the shoulder or arm.
- State clearly who you are. Speak in a normal tone of voice.
- Wait until your offer of assistance is accepted. Then listen to or ask for instructions.
- Treat adults as adults. Address people who have disabilities by their first names only when extending the same familiarity to all others.
- Do not lead the person without first asking; allow the person to hold your arm and control her or his own movements.
- Be prepared to repeat what you say, orally or in writing.
- Use positive phrases, such as "person with a developmental disability", rather than negative phrases, such as "mentally defective".

Touch and empathy

Empathy is the ability to understand what the patient is feeling and to respond appropriately. Acting empathically begins by recognizing any strong emotions the patient might be having. By recognizing these emotions, the patient care technician can give the patient the opportunity to talk about his feelings, as well as provide validation. Acting empathically allows the patient care technician to build trust and understanding with the patient.

Using touch is a nonverbal method of communicating with the patient. There are times when words are not enough to provide an adequate amount of comfort. In these times, holding a hand or giving a hug can do more to encourage conversation and provide comfort.

Providing information and self-disclosing

Providing information can be an effective tool in encouraging communication. When the patient is new to the health care facility, he may feel anxious about the unfamiliar surroundings. The patient care technician can help ease anxiety by providing the patient with information that is relevant to his care. However, the patient care technician must be careful not to provide specific information regarding the patient's diagnosis or test and lab results.

A patient care technician can also encourage communication by providing some information about herself in order to ease the patient's discomfort. However, the patient care technician must be careful not to dominate the conversation as the goal of therapeutic communication is to discover what the patient is thinking and feeling.

Communication block

A communication block is a statement or behavior that discourages therapeutic communication. A patient care technician may inadvertently use a communication block if she is hurried or is uncomfortable about the conversation at hand. Common communication blocks include the use of sarcasm or jokes in order to deflect the situation. The patient care technician may change the subject or may attempt to minimize the problem in order to ease her own discomfort. Offering false assurances or telling the patient how he should feel in a given situation may discourage the patient from communicating with the patient care technician.

Frequent use of the call bell

Frequent use of the call bell can occur for a number of reasons. The patient may not understand how to use the call bell or may push the wrong button accidentally. If this happens, a patient care technician can tape a piece of gauze over the button so that the patient can recognize the call button using his fingers. If using this method, it is important to check to make sure the call button can be pushed easily prior to leaving the room. Another reason that a patient may call frequently is that he is lonely. If this is the case, the patient care technician should make an effort to stop in to see the patient as frequently as possible. This may prevent frequent calls 'just to chat.' One way to prevent frequent use of the call bell is to make sure the patient has all necessary items within reach prior to leaving the room. Also, ask the patient if there is anything else he might need prior to leaving the room.

- 99 -

Communication with non-English speaking patients

Patients who are unable to speak English may be a challenge to communicate with. Though it is possible to ask a family member to aide in translating, many facilities prefer to use an official interpreter when conveying medically related information to the patient. Whether communicating through a family member or an interpreter, the patient care technician should look at the patient and address him while speaking. She should speak slowly and clearly, and watch the patient's body language and facial expressions closely as this can aide in the communication process. Before the family leaves, the patient care technician should ask them to write down a few common phrases, such as 'bathroom' and 'water,' to help with meeting the patient's needs.

Inability to communicate

Sometimes the patient care technician may be unable to communicate with the patient despite her best efforts. If the patient is intubated or has severe aphasia, he may not be able to effectively communicate his needs. The patient care technician should attempt to figure out what the patient is trying to say by running through a list of common needs, such as being thirsty, hot, cold, or in pain. If the patient care technician cannot figure out what the patient is trying to say, she should tell the patient that she is unable to understand him. She should not pretend to understand as this behavior can cause distress for the patient. The inability to communicate often results in frustration on the part of the patient. If this happens, the patient care technician should provide appropriate reassurance and emotional support.

Communication with the patient's family

Interaction with the patient's family can occur frequently during the course of patient care. The patient care technician can confer with the patient's family regarding procedures that are part of the patient care technician's scope of practice. When talking with the family while the patient is in the room, the patient care technician should make an effort to include the patient in the conversation; it is inappropriate to talk about the patient as if he is not there. The patient care technician cannot impart information about the patient's prognosis nor can she give information about test or lab results. If a family member has a question about the patient's care, he should be referred to the charge nurse.

A.M. and H.S. care

A.M. care is typically done in the morning, prior to any scheduled medical procedures. A.M. care involves a complete bath, shaving, dressing, hair care, oral care, and nails care, and may require changing of the bed linens. Hour of sleep (H.S.) care is done at bedtime. H.S. care involves an abbreviated form of skin care, including washing the patient's face and hands. Oral care should also be performed. A back rub may be given for 5 to 10 minutes to ensure the patient is relaxed and ready for sleep. Additional tasks may be performed, depending upon the patient's level of health and activity.

ADLs

Activities of daily living (ADLs) are tasks that are required to keep a person healthy and functional. Often, a person's level of health is determined by his ability to perform ADLs. The tasks are divided into two subgroups: basic ADLs and instrumental ADLs. Basic ADLs are tasks people must be perform in order to care for themselves. These include bathing, dressing, feeding, toileting, and walking. Instrumental ADLs are tasks performed in order to live independently within the community. These include shopping, cooking, housework, medication management, and money management.

Hygiene

The components of hygiene are the tasks that are necessary to promote patient health through cleanliness. These tasks include hair care, nail care, mouth care, bathing, and dressing. Hair care includes a gentle brushing and inspection of the patient's scalp. Nail care involves keeping the patient's nails trimmed and inspecting the patient's nail beds. Mouth care is performed to prevent tooth decay and to examine the patient's oral mucosa for sores or signs of infection. Bathing is done to keep the patient's skin clean and to inspect for lesions; this includes perineal care. The patient care technician must also ensure that dependent patients are able to dress and undress themselves properly.

Bathing

Over time, irritants can build on the patient's skin, which can cause a rash or skin breakdown. These irritants can also cause itching, which may provoke the patient to scratch the skin, creating a source of infection. Bathing cleanses the patient's skin of these irritants. Bathing can also promote patient relaxation and increase circulation. Bathing presents an opportunity to perform a thorough assessment of the patient's skin. Any signs of breakdown or lesions should be immediately reported. Furthermore, the patient's skin should be closely monitored for dryness, as this can cause cracking of the patient's skin.

A tub bath is preferred when the patient is strong enough to get into and out of the bathtub. It involves completely washing the patient, including performing perineal care. A tub bath can be given daily. However, if the patient's skin is showing signs of dryness, the frequency may be reduced to two or three times a week. A bed bath is given to a patient when he is unable to ambulate. A complete bed bath involves cleansing the patient's skin and changing the patient's linens. If the patient is incontinent of urine or stool, a partial bath may be given. This involves cleansing only those parts of the body that have been soiled and changing only those linens that are dirty.

Tub bath

Prior to beginning the tub bath, wash your hands, greet the patient, and explain what you are going to do. Make sure the bathtub has been cleaned. Place towels in the tub and on the floor outside the tub to prevent slipping. Ambulate the patient to the tub, observing all precautions. Once the patient is in the tub, fill it to the desired level. Make sure the water temperature is about 115 degrees. Provide privacy while the patient washes, but maintain close supervision to make sure the patient does not slip. Wash the patient's back and any area he is unable to reach. Drain the water, and dry the patient. Assist the patient into a standing position, and carefully help him out of the tub. Assist the patient in putting on his clothes. Position the patient for comfort, clean the tub, and wash your hands.

<u>Bed bath</u>

A bed bath can be a time-consuming procedure, depending upon the patient's level of activity. One way to facilitate a bed bath is to make sure that all of the necessary supplies are present prior to starting the bath. A patient care technician will require a basin of water, soap, lotion, and baby powder. The water should be warmed to between 105 and 115 degrees. The patient care technician will need several washcloths and at least two towels. The patient care technician should also have a pair of gloves to wear while giving the bath. Linens should be changed while the bed bath is being performed. In order to change the bed, the patient care technician will need a fitted sheet, a bed pad, a flat sheet, a blanket, and pillowcases.

Prior to beginning the bed bath, wash your hands, greet the patient, and explain what you are going to do. Fill a basin with water at a temperature of between 105 and 115 degrees, and remove as much medical equipment as possible. Keep the patient covered to maintain dignity. Allow the patient to bathe as much of himself as possible. Begin by washing the patient's face, moving downward to the arms, the chest, abdomen, legs, back, and perineal area. Use a different washcloth for each area of the body. If necessary, change the patient's bed linens while washing the back. Apply lotion if desired. After the bath has been completed, reposition the patient for comfort and wash your hands.

<u>Perineal care</u>

Perineal care is an important part of bathing because it allows the patient care technician to inspect the skin of the perineal area. If done properly, it also decreases the risk for urinary tract infections. Perineal care should be done during a complete bath and should also be performed after the patient is incontinent. Wash your hands, and don a pair of gloves. Instruct the patient to open his legs. Cleanse the skin of the perineal area, using front to back movements. Never wash from back to front as this can introduce germs from the anus to the urethral area. After the skin has been cleansed, completely dry the area. Do not reuse the linens used to wash the peri area. Obtain a clean towel and washcloth to finish the bath.

Hair care

Hair care is a procedure that helps to improve patient comfort and morale. It stimulates blood circulation within the scalp. Hair washing also removes excess oils and bacteria. Frequency of hair care depends upon the amount of oil that has accumulated in the patient's hair, as well as the level of dryness of the scalp. The patient care technician must be vigilant while performing hair care. Head lice, an excessive amount of dandruff, or sores on the scalp should be reported to the nurse immediately if noticed by the patient care technician. Such findings may require special precautions to be taken while performing hair care in the future.

Prior to beginning hair care on the patient, wash your hands, greet the patient, and explain what you are going to do. Don a pair of gloves. Raise the head of the bed to a comfortable level, and place a towel beneath the patient's head. Part the patient's hair into manageable sections, and run the comb or brush slowly through it. If the hair is tangled, hold the strand of hair above the tangle while combing it to prevent pulling the patient's hair. As you are combing, carefully inspect the scalp for any lesions, lice, or signs of dryness. Try to shape the hair into the patient's preferred style; even parting the hair on the correct side can provide a greater level of comfort for the patient. After hair care is complete, remove the towel and reposition the patient for comfort.

Shaving a patient

Prior to beginning the procedure, wash your hands, greet the patient, and explain what you are going to do. Apply a pair of gloves, and use a wet washcloth to moisten the hair on the patient's face and neck. Check the razor to make sure it does not have any loose blades or jagged edges. Drape the patient with a towel, and apply shaving cream to the area that needs to be shaved. Use one hand to pull the skin taut, while moving the razor with firm strokes in the direction that the hair is growing. Rinse the razor in a basin of water as often as necessary. Use a moistened washcloth to rinse off all remaining shaving cream.

Oral care

Some patients may be unable to perform oral care on themselves as a result of palsy or weakness in the upper extremities. Before beginning oral care, wash your hands, greet the patient, and explain what you are going to do. Don a pair of gloves, and drape a towel over the patient. Raise the level of the bed to a comfortable height, and position the head of the bed greater than 30 degrees. Using a toothbrush, thoroughly clean the patient's teeth, gums, and tongue. While performing oral care, carefully inspect the patient's mouth for any lesions or signs of infection. If the patient is able to take small amounts of water without aspirating, allow him to rinse his mouth and spit the water into an emesis basin. Position the patient for comfort, and wash your hands.

Unconscious patient
Prior to beginning oral care on an unconscious patient, wash your hands, check the patient's name band, and explain what you are going to do. Don a pair of gloves, and drape a towel over the patient's chest. Adjust the level of the bed to a comfortable height, and raise the head of the bed greater than 30 degrees. Turn the patient's head toward you, and hold the mouth open with a tongue depressor in one hand. Clean the patient's teeth, gums, and tongue. After cleaning has been completed, suction the secretions out of the patient's mouth. Position the patient for comfort, remove the gloves, and wash your hands.

Denture care
Prior to beginning denture care, wash your hands, greet the patient, and explain what you are going to do. Don a pair of gloves, and obtain the patient's dentures. Place a towel or washcloth in the sink to prevent breakage if the dentures are accidentally dropped. Using a toothbrush, clean the surface of the patient's dentures. Place them in a denture cup filled with cool water. Provide oral care to the patient using sponge swabs and mouthwash; carefully observe for any lesions or signs of infection. After the procedure has been completed, position the patient for comfort and wash your hands.

Abnormal findings
Performing oral care presents an ideal opportunity to examine the patient's oral mucosa for abnormalities. The patient care technician should carefully observe the patient's mouth for any sores, redness, or bleeding on the patient's lips or gums. Cracking may occur on the patient's lips as a result of dryness. The patient care technician should also be observant for any odor that may occur as a result of infection. Thrush is a fungal infection that can develop as a result of poor oral care or after taking certain medications. If thrush is present,

the patient may appear with white patches covering the tongue or gums. The patient may also complain of a thick, furry feeling in the mouth.

Nail care

Nail care is important for a number of reasons. The primary purpose of nail care is to remove bacteria and dirt from the patient's nail beds, preventing the spread of microorganisms. Appropriate nail care also ensures the patient's nails are not sharp or jagged, which increases the risk of infection from breakage of the skin. While performing nail care, the patient care technician has the opportunity to inspect the patient's nail beds for any signs of inflammation or fungal growth. Any signs of infection or discoloration should immediately be reported to the nurse.

Prior to beginning nail care, wash your hands, greet the patient, and explain what you are going to do. Don a pair of gloves. Soak the patient's hands in warm water to soften them and prevent the nails from cracking. Carefully remove any dirt from beneath the patient's nails. Trim each nail by cutting straight across with a pair of nail clippers, then round the edges using an emery board. Be careful not to cut the nails too short as this may cause irritation to the nail bed. If desired, apply lotion to the patient's nails. After nail care has been completed, reposition the patient for comfort and wash your hands.

A patient care technician should exercise caution when providing nail care to patients who are receiving anticoagulation therapy as this type of medication puts the patient at an increased risk for bleeding. Nail care should not be performed on patients with a history of diabetes or decreased circulation in their feet. Diabetes and low circulation affect the ability of the tissue to repair itself. As a result, even the smallest cut on the skin places the patient at risk for severe ulcers on the feet. Prior to performing nail care, the patient care technician should check the facility policies to ensure that nail cutting falls within her scope of practice.

Back rub

Prior to giving a backrub, wash your hands, greet the patient, and explain what you are going to do. Ensure that privacy is provided, and don a pair of gloves. If necessary, wash the patient's back with warm water and dry it completely. Warm the lotion in the basin of water, and apply a small amount to your hands. Begin the backrub at the small of the patient's back, and work your way toward the shoulders using long, firm strokes. Use a circular motion when rubbing over bony areas to prevent irritating the skin. While performing the backrub, carefully observe the patient's skin for any signs of breakdown. After the back rub has been completed, position the patient for comfort and wash your hands.

Bedpan

Wash your hands, and greet the patient. Explain what you are going to do. Make sure the patient has privacy, and put on a pair of gloves. Lay the patient flat in a supine position, and turn him on his side. Place the bedpan over the buttocks, and carefully roll him back onto his back. Instruct the patient to open his legs, and make sure the bedpan has been placed properly. Raise the head of the bed, give the patient the call bell, and instruct the patient to call when finished. Remove your gloves, and wash your hands. When the patient is ready to get off the bedpan, once again ensure the patient has privacy. Wash your hands, and don a

- 104 -

pair of gloves. Lay the head of the bed flat, and turn the patient on his side. While turning the patient, support the bedpan in order to prevent secretions from leaking into the bed. Remove the bedpan, and set it to one side. Provide perineal care for the patient. Position the patient for comfort, and allow him to wash his hands with a damp rag, if desired. Measure the output, and dispose of the secretions.

Feeding assistance

The amount of feeding assistance that should be provided depends upon the individual patient. Some patients will not require assistance to feed themselves. If the patient is able to feed himself, he should be allowed to do so to encourage independence. Some assistance may be required, such as cutting larger portions and opening beverages. Some patients, such as those who suffer from blindness, may only need verbal cues to eat.
Some patients are unable to feed themselves as a result of weakness or paralysis of the upper body. These patients will require their food be cut and each bite fed to them. Patient care technicians should be careful to take their time and not rush the feeding. They should ensure the patient has chewed and swallowed every bite, before offering the next bit of food.

Before taking the tray into the patient's room, the patient care technician should check to make sure the patient is receiving the correct tray. Check the patient's armband and compare it to the name and room number on the tray. Check to make sure the patient's tray contains foods that are appropriate for the patient's ordered diet. Wash your hands, raise the head of the patient's bed, and place a towel over him to prevent bits of food from falling into bed. Explain to the patient what foods are being served on the tray, and allow the patient to select what foods he will be fed first. If the patient requires further assistance, cut any large pieces of food into bite-size pieces and open any containers. When providing a bite to the patient, ensure the spoon is only half full. Use only the tip of the spoon to feed him. Feed the patient slowly, ensuring the patient has swallowed all of the food in his mouth before offering the next bite. Make sure the patient has had enough food to eat before taking the tray away. If the patient appears to be having difficulty swallowing, stop feeding the patient immediately and notify the nurse.

After the patient has finished eating, remove the meal tray and calculate the amount of food the patient took in. If the patient is on a calorie count diet, calculate the percentage of food eaten and tolerance to the food. If the patient's intake and output is being monitored, calculate the amount of fluid the patient took in. Report these findings to the nurse. Position the patient for comfort, and place the call light within reach. Make sure any necessary items, such as the tray table and personal items, are within reach. Hand hygiene should then be performed.

Clock method of feeding

The clock method is a way of describing the placement of food on a plate to a visually impaired patient who is able to feed himself. The patient should be instructed to picture the plate as a clock face, with positions of food located at corresponding numbers. For example, the meat can be at the 12 o'clock position, the vegetables at the 3 o'clock position, bread at the 6 o'clock position, and the fruit at the 9 o'clock position. The patient care technician should try to repeat this pattern at every meal so that the patient is familiar with the locations of each type of food.

Meeting special dietary needs

Upon admission to the hospital or long-term care facility, the patient care technician should make note of any cultural or religious requests that the patient may have regarding dietary needs. The facility dietary service should be notified as soon as possible to ensure the patient is provided with appropriate foods. Prior to taking the tray in to the room, the patient care technician should check to make sure the food on the tray meets the patient's dietary restrictions. If it does not, the dietary service should be notified regarding the problem, and a replacement meal should be obtained as soon as possible.

Therapeutic diets

NPO, clear liquid, and mechanical soft
NPO (nothing by mouth) is a diet that is ordered for patients who are not allowed to eat. It is typically ordered in anticipation of medical testing or a surgical procedure. Patient status will also be made NPO if it is unsafe for the individual to eat, such as a patient who is intubated, sedated, or unable to swallow properly. A clear liquid diet is the first diet prescribed after a patient is taken off NPO status. It is typically ordered to allow the patient to eat without experiencing nausea. A mechanical soft diet is prescribed for patients who have difficulty chewing, such as patients who do not have their dentures. It is also intended to help patients to transition from NPO to a regular diet.

Regular, calorie count, low sodium, and cardiac
The diet that is prescribed for a patient depends upon the individual's health history. A regular diet has no dietary restrictions; patients can eat whatever they like. A calorie count diet is typically ordered for diabetic patients; it limits the amount of sugar the patient takes in and counts the number of calories and carbohydrates the patient consumes. A low-sodium diet is prescribed to limit the amount of salt ingested by patients with a history of renal impairment or hypertension. A cardiac diet is ordered for patients with a history of cardiac problems; while on this diet, they are served low-fat, low-calorie, and low-sodium foods.

Nutrients

Nutrients are elements in nature that are necessary in order to live. Our bodies absorb the nutrients from the foods we eat. Nutrients are divided into six groups: carbohydrates, proteins, fats, minerals, vitamins, and water. Carbohydrates are composed primarily of sugar and serve as the main source of energy. Protein is made primarily of amino acids and aids in tissue repair. Fats are composed of fatty acids and are essential for cell membrane integrity and thermal regulation. Minerals and vitamins are needed to aid metabolism and a number of other body processes. Water acts as a solvent and is also required for a number of body processes.

Nutrients necessary for blood production

Humans need the nutrients iron, folate, Vitamin B_6 Vitamin B12, Vitamin C, Vitamin E, Vitamin K, riboflavin, copper, zinc, and protein to manufacture blood in the bone marrow. Even if these nutrients are adequate, the patient cannot produce sufficient blood without the hormone erythropoietin from the kidneys. Therefore, patients with end-stage renal failure who are on dialysis become anemic.

Anemia

Anemia is lack of blood or a deficiency in red blood cells. Signs and symptoms of anemia are fatigue, thirst, rapid pulse, pallor, dizziness, sweating, shortness of breath, abdominal or chest pain, leg cramps, and syncope. Aplastic anemia results from suppressed bone marrow, due to leukemia, radiation or poisoning. Protein deficiency causes kwashiorkor anemia. Strict vegetarianism and chronic bleeding (e.g., heavy menstruation) deplete iron stores (ferritin), thereby causing iron deficiency anemia. Vitamin B12 deficiency causes pernicious anemia. Anemia occurs from increased red blood cell destruction from sickle-cell anemia, thalassemia, G6PD deficiency, autoimmune reaction, inherited disorders, hemolytic poison, or an enlarged spleen.

Fat-soluble vitamins

Vitamin A (retinol) aids growth, development, immune function, and maintains night vision. Sources are butter, egg yolks, cod liver oil, yellow and green leafy vegetables, and prunes. Deficiency causes night blindness, poor visual acuity, skin disorders, and bronchopulmonary dysplasia in low birth weight newborns. Vitamin D (calciferol) aids calcium & phosphorus absorption for bone and teeth formation and necessary for normal growth and development. Sources are milk, cod liver oil, butter, and egg yolks. Sunlight activates Vitamin D. Deficiency causes rickets and osteomalacia (soft bones, bowed legs) and dental caries. Vitamin E (tocopherols) is an antioxidant found in sunflower seeds, wheat germ, egg yolks, vegetable oils, almonds, olives, and papaya. Deficiency causes hemolytic anemia of premature newborns. Vitamin K (quinones) is a necessary for normal clotting of the blood and is found in green leafy vegetables, meat, dairy products, alfalfa, fishmeal, oats, wheat, and rye. Deficiency causes hemorrhagic disease of the newborn. Caution must be taken if anticoagulants are being used as this may affect how the clotting of the blood. There is no known toxicity. The small intestine absorbs fat-soluble vitamins, so patients who have had bowel resections, cystic fibrosis or malabsorption may have deficiencies. Fat-soluble vitamins accumulate in fat and the liver, and can be toxic.

Food pyramid

The food guide pyramid was published by the U.S. Department of Agriculture to educate the public on the recommended daily nutrition requirements. It is visualized by five angled strips that form the shape of a pyramid. The first strip symbolizes the grains group, which includes rice, bread, and pasta. The second strip symbolizes vegetables. The third strip symbolizes fruit. The fourth strip symbolizes milk and cheese. The fifth strip symbolizes meat and beans. The food pyramid recommends serving sizes measured in ounces, with the size of the serving dependent upon the patient's age and gender.

Difficulty swallowing

A helpless patient is at a significant risk for aspirating food. During aspiration, small amounts of food and water move down the trachea and into the patient's lungs. Forceful coughing or a wet-sounding voice after swallowing a bite of food may be an indication of aspiration. If a patient needs to chew food for long periods of time or requires multiple attempts to swallow food, he may be aspirating. Other indications include unusual head movements while trying to swallow, difficulty breathing, drooling while eating, or pocketing food in the cheeks. All of these signs should be reported to the patient's nurse.

Hydration

Water is a vitally important nutrient. It aids in metabolism, temperature regulation, and elimination of body waste. Water is constantly lost through normal sweating, elimination, and exhalation. Certain states, such as illness and increased activity, can cause increased water loss. It is recommended that the patient take in at least 1500cc to 2000cc or 8 to 10 glasses of water every day to maintain hydration and replace lost body fluids. If the patient does not receive an adequate amount of fluids, dehydration may occur. If left uncorrected, dehydration can be a fatal condition.

Applying anti-embolism stockings

Prior to applying anti-embolism stockings, wash your hands, greet the patient, and explain what you are going to do. Verify the anti-embolism stockings are the proper size for the patient based upon height and weight; they should be tight without cutting off circulation. Place the patient in a supine position. Gather the fabric of the anti-embolism stocking and slide it onto the patient's foot. Roll the stocking upward until the upper edge is placed above the patient's knee. Check to make sure there are no wrinkles in the stocking and that the stocking is placed properly so that the toes and heels are in the appropriate spots. Once the stocking is in place, position the patient for comfort, remove your gloves, and wash your hands.

Applying elastic bandages

Prior to applying an elastic bandage, check the order to confirm where the bandage is to be placed. Wash your hands, greet the patient, and explain what you are going to do. Apply a pair of gloves. Hold the end of the bandage in place with one hand, and wrap it around the extremity twice to secure it. Continue to wrap the bandage around the area that needs to be covered, working from bottom to top. While wrapping, overlap the bandages to keep them from sliding down and to ensure the area is covered. Once the elastic bandage is in place, secure it with tape, clips, or Velcro. Remove the gloves, and wash your hands.

Monitoring patients with elastic bandages or anti-embolism stockings

While patients are wearing anti-embolism stockings or elastic bandages, it is important to monitor them closely to ensure they receive an appropriate amount of circulation to their extremities. Frequently assess the patient's toes (or fingers, if the elastic bandage is on the arm) to check for signs of decreased circulation. Any complaints of numbness, tingling, or decreased sensation in the extremity should be reported to the nurse and investigated immediately. Make sure to remove the patient's anti-embolism stockings every 8 hours to allow for circulation. Elastic bandages should be removed per the doctor's order.

Range of motion exercises

Patients who are bed bound are at an increased risk of muscle deterioration from lack of use. Lack of regular exercise also places patients at risk for developing contractures, a painful condition that results in the permanent shortening of the muscle or tendon. Range-of-motion exercises can be performed to maintain muscle tone during periods in which the patient lacks the strength to perform other forms of activity. Patients may also be assisted with performing range-of-motion activities if they are unable to do so themselves, such as in cases in which patients are sedated or comatose.

Range-of-motion exercises are typically performed during the patient's bath. They can be performed while the patient is sitting in a chair or lying in bed. Each exercise should be performed 10 times to ensure it is effective. Wash your hands, and explain to the patient what you are going to do. Raise the level of the bed until it is a comfortable height for you. Begin by performing range-of-motion exercises on the patient's head; instruct the patient to rotate his head from one side to the other. This exercise should not be performed on patients who have suffered neck or spinal cord injuries. Work on the arms next. Flex and extend both arms at the elbow, then abduct and adduct the arm. Flex and extend both wrists and all fingers. Range of motion of the legs includes flexion and extension of the leg at the knee, as well as abduction and adduction of the leg. Finally, flex and extend the ankles and toes.

Range-of-motion exercises should be performed at least once or twice every day to make sure the patient's joints do not become contracted. Stiffness or the inability to move the joint may be an indication of the onset of contractures; if either of these symptoms is noticed, they should be reported to the nurse immediately. While performing range of motion, the patient care technician should monitor for any signs of swelling or inflammation in the joints. If the patient experiences sudden severe pain or respiratory distress while performing range of motion, the nurse should be notified immediately.

AROM and PROM
Active range of motion (AROM) occurs when patients are able to perform range-of-motion activities by themselves. Though they may receive directions from the patient care technician, patients perform the bulk of the exercise. Passive range of motion (PROM) consists of the same exercises that are performed during AROM. PROM occurs when the patient care technician is performing range-of-motion activities on a sedated or comatose patient to prevent muscle weakness. PROM may also be performed on patients whose muscle weakness is so pronounced that they require assistance in order to perform the activity.

Flexion, extension, abduction, adduction, and rotation
Flexion refers to bending at a joint, resulting in a decrease in the angle of the joint. Extension refers to the straightening of a joint, or increasing the angle of that joint. For example, when the arm is bent at the elbow, it is flexed. When the arm is straightened, it is extended. Abduction refers to the movement away from the trunk. Adduction refers to a movement that brings a limb closer to the trunk. When the arm is moved away from the body, such as during jumping jacks, it is abducted. When it moves back toward the body, it is adducted. Rotation occurs when a part of the body pivots on a central axis. When the head turns from side to side, it is considered to be rotating.

Preventing skin irritation

Skin irritation can result in sores and infection. There are a number of measures a patient care technician can take to prevent skin irritation from occurring. One way to avoid skin rash or irritation is to completely cleanse the skin of any urine or feces if the patient has soiled himself. Because urine and stool is acidic in nature, skin breakdown can occur quickly if left close to the patient's skin. If the patient is incontinent, applying water resistant lotion will protect the skin by creating a barrier that will prevent rashes or breakdown. Frequent repositioning should also be performed to prevent skin breakdown. A bedridden patient should be turned every two hours to prevent breakdown over bony prominences.

Dressing a dependent patient

When the patient has suffered a stroke, it can result in weakness on one side of the patient's body. Often, the patient may require assistance in daily activities, such as dressing. It is important to teach the patient how to clothe himself safely to promote independence and decrease the risk of falling. Before beginning to assist the patient in undressing, make sure the clean set of clothes is within easy reach. When removing clothing, the patient should be taught to undress the weakened side first. For example, a patient with weakness on the right side should remove the right arm from the sleeve first. When putting clean clothes on, the patient should be taught to dress the strong side first.

Patients with visual impairment

A patient care technician should take special precautions when caring for a patient who has a visual impairment. Prior to interacting with the patient, the patient care technician should acquaint herself with the type of visual impairment the patient has. She should make sure to identify herself as soon as she enters the room and stand within the patient's visual field while interacting with him. While ambulating the patient, the patient care technician should allow the patient to move as freely as possible and provide clear verbal cues regarding potential obstacles. The furniture in the patient's room should not be moved to allow the patient to become familiar with the surroundings.

Alleviating symptoms of Sundowner's syndrome

There are a number of steps a patient care technician can take to decrease the severity of Sundowner's syndrome. In the morning, the patient care technician should open the curtains and blinds and allow the patient to see outside to reorient them to time of day. Encourage exercise during the day. Plan all strenuous activities for the morning so that there is an adequate amount of time to relax prior to bedtime. Do not allow the patient to sleep during the day as this will make it difficult to sleep during the night. Plan a few relaxing activities before bed, such as therapeutic massage or quiet reading time. These activities should be performed at the same time every night to establish a routine. When it is time to sleep, darken the room as much as possible to further reinforce time of day.

Hearing impaired patient

If the patient has difficulty hearing in one ear, the patient care technician should talk while standing on the side that the patient can hear. The patient care technician should introduce herself and speak slowly and clearly. The patient care technician should face the patient while talking to give him the opportunity to read lips. While talking to the patient, the patient care technician should try to limit background noise and deepen the tone of her voice in order to make herself better heard. If the patient can see well, communication can be achieved using written messages rather than speaking.

Caring for a patient with aphasia

Prior to interacting with the patient, the patient care technician should acquaint herself with the type of aphasia the patient has and communicate with the patient accordingly. The key to caring for a patient with aphasia is to avoid becoming frustrated. Do not rush the patient; allow him time to gather his thoughts and say what he is trying to say. Avoid attempting to speak for the patient. Try to use a picture or letter board to assist with communication. If possible, allow the patient to write messages in order to communicate.

Care for a patient with contractures

There are a number of treatment options for a patient with contractures. When a patient first develops a contracture, the nurse and the physical therapist should be notified. Attempts should be made to mobilize the joint using range-of-motion techniques. Heat therapy may be used prior to initiating activity to ease pain and increase flexibility. In some cases, the affected joint may be placed in a splint, which will continuously stretch the joint. Care of the splint should be performed as ordered by the doctor. If the contracture does not respond to other treatments, the patient may be taken to surgery to manipulate the tendon.

Preventing edema

Edema can develop in the patient's extremities as a result of fluid overload or inactivity. The patient care technician can prevent swelling by encouraging the patient to move. If the patient is unable to walk, range-of-motion exercises should be frequently performed. While in bed or in the chair, the patient's legs should be elevated on pillows to prevent swelling in the lower extremities. Massaging the patient's extremities using lotion can also prevent edema. If the patient has a history of heart or kidney failure, his fluid and sodium intake should be closely monitored as too much can result in increased edema.

Caring for a confused patient

Confusion that develops in the hospital or extended-care facility is typically a symptom of a physiological problem. If the patient care technician notices confusion in a patient who was previously oriented, the nurse should be notified immediately. The patient care technician should try to find out what the patient's normal orientation was prior to entering the hospital; this can be done by reviewing records and talking to family members. The patient care technician should be observant for any signs of the physiological problem that may be causing the confusion. For example, cloudy urine may indicate a urinary tract infection, which could result in confusion in the elderly. Until the cause of the confusion is determined, the patient care technician should provide a safe, non-threatening environment while attempting to reorient the patient to the surroundings.

Caring for an agitated patient

When a patient becomes agitated, the key is to remain calm. Remind the patient who you are, and attempt to reorient the patient to the surroundings. Speak calmly and clearly; attempt to learn what it is that is causing the patient to become agitated. Treat the patient as you want him to behave. While talking to the patient, assume a non-threatening posture. If possible, enlist the aid of family members to calm the patient down. If all of these

Copyright © Mometrix Media. You have been licensed one copy of this document for personal use only. Any other reproduction or redistribution is strictly prohibited. All rights reserved.

measures fail and the patient is behaving in a way that may cause harm to himself or to other people, restraints may be required.

Reality orientation

Reality orientation is a set of activities that are performed with a confused patient in an attempt to reorient him to his environment. The first step of reality orientation is to approach the patient in a friendly, non-threatening manner. While interacting with the patient, the patient care technician should provide verbal reminders regarding time and place. The patient care technician should provide the patient with physical reminders of the surroundings, such as writing the date on a whiteboard within the patient's visual field or showing the patient where a clock can be located.

Affect of culture on outlook

Culture is defined as the behavior and belief systems of a particular group. A person's cultural outlook is shaped by ethnicity, gender, and age. It affects his outlook on all things, including health care. It can affect the types of foods the patient might eat while sick, his behaviors during illness, and his attitude about death and dying. The patient's cultural beliefs should be taken into account when planning care. If the patient's cultural beliefs are not taken into account, it may increase the patient's stress level, hindering the healing process.

Considerations with Muslim patients

It is important to ask the patient if he has any specific dietary restrictions. Many strict practicing Muslims will eat only specially slaughtered fish, chicken, and beef. Most Muslims will not eat pork products. Try to avoid handing a Muslim patient anything with the left hand as that is the hand that is reserved for performing perineal care on oneself. Muslims place a strong emphasis on cleanliness. Many Muslims prefer to wash with soap and water after using the bedpan, rather than using toilet paper. They should also be provided with fresh water to wash with prior to their prayers. If possible, female patients should be cared for by female patient care technicians.

Considerations with Christian patients

It is important for the patient care technician to ask if the patient has any dietary restrictions. Though most Christians do not have dietary restrictions as a result of their faith, some may have self-imposed dietary restrictions. Some Catholic patients may wish to fast during Lent. During their stay, some Catholic or Orthodox Christian patients may choose to receive communion or give confession during their hospitalization. Some patients may request to receive Last Rites if they are critically ill or dying. It is important to notify the charge nurse immediately if the patient requests to see a priest during his stay. In many cases, the patient or family will know a priest they would want to call.

Considerations with Hindu patients

It is important for the patient care technician to inquire about any specific dietary needs. Most Hindus are vegetarian or vegan; even those that do eat meat may refuse to eat beef or pork. After using the bedpan, most Hindu patients prefer to wash their perineal area using clean water rather than using toilet paper. The patient care technician should make it available if requested. Some Hindus may prefer to wash in the shower rather than sitting in the bath. Members of the Hindu faith particularly value privacy; if possible, the patient should be cared for by a patient care technician who is of the same gender. Some Hindu patients may prefer to die while lying on the ground to maintain closeness between the individual and Mother Earth. If necessary, a Hindu priest may be called in to perform holy rites for the patient.

Considerations with Jewish patients

Orthodox Jews eat only kosher meat and typically avoid dishes in which milk and meat have been prepared together. Other types of foods that are forbidden include pork products, meat from birds of prey, and shellfish. Most Jewish patients prefer to wash their hands and say a brief prayer prior to eating; the patient care technician should provide them with an opportunity to do so. Jewish men may prefer to remain bearded or may choose to shave using an electric razor rather than a razor blade. Jewish patients observe specific practices regarding death. The family will notify their Synagogue of the patient's impending death; if there is no family present, the health care staff should do so. After the death, three members of the family typically wash the body. Burial should take place within 24 hours after dying.

Considerations with Mormon patients

Many Mormons follow a set of dietary restrictions put forward in the *Word of Wisdom*. It teaches against the use of stimulants, such as coffee, tea, and other caffeinated beverages. Though most Mormons are not strict vegetarians, they do tend to eat meat sparingly. Some Mormons may wear a special undergarment that should be treated with the utmost privacy. It can be removed for laundering and washing but is otherwise worn at all times. Though Mormons do not have specific rites or rituals regarding a dying patient, the patient care technician should make sure to allow the family to spend as much time as possible with the patient in his final hours. If the patient wears the sacred undergarment, it should be put back on the body after postmortem care has been performed.

Considerations with Buddhist patients

It is important for a patient care technician to inquire about a Buddhist's dietary needs on admission as many Buddhist patients are vegetarians or vegans. Many Buddhists fast on specific days, including the days of the New Moon and Full Moon. On fasting days, a Buddhist will only eat at specific times. The patient care technician should collaborate with the patient on these days to ensure he gets his meal tray at appropriate times.
The type of rituals surrounding death and dying varies depending on the patient's traditions. The patient may request a Buddhist monk or nun to perform chants in order to assist in the patient's passing. If possible, the body should not be touched until 3 to 8 hours after death before preparing the body for death.

Intake and output measurement

Intake and output (I&O) is an important indicator of fluid balance. Intake is calculated by measuring all of the fluid the patient drinks. Output is calculated by measuring all of the fluid the patient secretes, including urine, stool, and emesis. All measurements should be recorded in cubic centimeters (cc). Calculating I&O over a period of a few days can give an indication of the patient's fluid status. Ideally, intake should equal output. If intake exceeds output, then the patient may be fluid overloaded. If output exceeds intake, the patient may be dehydrated.

Measuring intake

In order to measure a patient's intake, the patient care technician must measure any liquids the patient takes in over a 24-hour period. This includes any water, milk, and juice the patient might drink, as well as any foods that melt at room temperature, such as ice cream, pudding, or jello. While measuring intake, the patient care technician should also include any tube feeding or any fluid that is used to flush a nasogastric tube. If the patient is receiving IV therapy, all IV fluids and medications suspended in IV fluid should be included in the patient's total intake. IV intake should also include any IV fluids that the patient received during surgery. Intake should be calculated in cubic centimeters (cc) and added up over a 24-hour period. That total should then be reported to the nurse.

Observations regarding bowel movements

After the patient moves his bowels, the patient care technician should make careful note of the color and character of the stool. If the patient has multiple bouts of diarrhea, the nurse should be notified as this places the patient at risk of developing dehydration. Dark, tarry stools indicate the patient may be bleeding within the intestinal tract. Frank blood should also be reported. Furthermore, if the patient has not had a bowel movement in more than three days, the nurse should be notified as this places the patient at risk for developing constipation.

Measuring output

Output measures the amount of fluid the patient excretes during a 24-hour period. All urine should be measured prior to being discarded. The amount of liquid stool in a bedpan should be estimated prior to being discarded. If the patient has a nasogastric tube to wall suction, the patient care technician should note how much drainage the patient has had out of the tube. If the patient has a wound that is hooked to suction, note how much blood has been removed from the wound. If the patient is having drainage out of a wound that is not to suction, the patient care technician should note how many times the dressing needs to be changed. Estimated blood loss from surgery should also be included as output. Add all secretions over a 24-hour period, and make a note of it on the patient's chart.

Calculating intake and output

After intake and output have been calculated over a 24-hour period, the two numbers should be compared. Ideally, intake should equal output as this indicates an equal fluid balance. Too much intake puts the patient at a risk for fluid overload, while too much output puts the patient at risk for dehydration. After comparing intake and output over a 24-hour period, the patient care technician should compare intake and output over the past few days. This gives a better indication of the patient's ongoing fluid status. For example, a high intake on one day may be compensated on the following day with a high output, placing the patient's fluid balance at an equal level.

Encouraging fluid intake

If a patient is dehydrated, he must increase the amount of fluids that he consumes in order to restore fluid balance. Explain to the patient why it is important to consume more fluids, and make sure a water pitcher and glass is within reach. Fluids should be encouraged each time you go into the patient's room. Also, make other fluids available, such as fruit juice or decaffeinated tea or coffee. Try to avoid sugary sodas or caffeinated beverages as these may not quench the patient's thirst. If the patient has family present, ask them to also encourage the patient to drink more.

Caring for a constipated patient

During hospitalization, there is a strong risk that the patient will develop constipation. This is often the result of decreased activity and the administration of medications that reduce gastrointestinal motility. The patient's bowel habits should be closely monitored. If the patient is using a bedpan, the consistency, color, and amount of stool should be noted after every bowel movement. If the patient is able to go to the bathroom without assistance, the patient care technician should inquire about the quality and frequency of the patient's stools. If the patient is constipated, it is important to encourage fluids to prevent drying of the stool. Warm liquids and juices are particularly effective in improving gastrointestinal motility. Caffeinated beverages should be avoided. Foods that are high in fiber should also be encouraged.

Caring for a patient with diarrhea

Patients who experience multiple bouts of diarrhea are at a significant risk for developing dehydration. They should be closely monitored for any signs or symptoms of dehydration. The number of stools and amount of fluid that are passed should be monitored. A stool specimen should be collected as soon as possible to determine the cause of the diarrhea. If the patient is having frequent diarrhea, it is important to encourage him to drink fluids to prevent him from becoming dehydrated. If his diet allows, the patient should be encouraged to drink two glasses of fluid for every bout of diarrhea. Proper hand hygiene should also be encouraged.

Preventing urinary tract infection

There are a number of ways that a urinary tract infection can be prevented. If a patient's diet tolerates it, oral fluids should be encouraged. Cranberry juice is particularly helpful in preventing urinary tract infections because it raises the acidity of the urine. If the patient needs assistance to void, help him to the bathroom as soon as possible as holding in urine can increase the patient's risk for developing an infection. While performing perineal care, the patient care technician should make sure to wash female patients from front to back. If the patient is able to ambulate, showers should be encouraged rather than baths.

Preventing pressure sores

There are a number of methods available to prevent the formation of pressure sores. The primary method of prevention is frequent repositioning. The patient should be turned and repositioned at least every two hours to prevent skin breakdown. Pillows may be used to provide additional support. The patient's feet should be elevated to prevent breakdown on the ankles, and the head of the bed should be kept at less than a 30-degree angle to reduce pressure on the buttocks. The patient's skin should be assessed frequently. The patient's nutritional status should be closely monitored as well since patients who have poor nutrition are at an increased risk of developing a pressure sore.

<u>Air mattress and egg crate mattress</u>
Pressure ulcers typically develop when the patient is unable to move as a result of illness or injury. As the patient lies in bed, his weight causes breakdown over bony prominences, such as over the shoulder blades and coccyx. When inflated, an air mattress decreases the amount of pressure placed upon the bony prominences. An egg crate mattress is a foam cushion that has alternating raised areas and grooves that decrease the area of pressure on bony prominences. Though these items do not replace turning the patient, they can aid in preventing pressure sores in high-risk patients.

Pressure sore treatment

Pressure sores are difficult to heal as a result of the patient's compromised health status. If a patient develops a pressure sore, it is important to ensure it does not get worse by frequently turning and repositioning the patient. The patient should be placed on a support surface, such as an air mattress. This helps to decrease the amount of pressure on bony prominences. The skin over the affected area should be kept clean and dry. Dressings can be applied to the pressure sore, though the type of dressing depends on the severity of the pressure ulcer. It is also important to ensure the patient maintains good nutrition to ensure healing.

Transferring a patient from bed to wheelchair

Care must be taken while transferring a patient from the bed to the wheelchair to prevent falling during the transfer. Prior to moving the patient, make sure the bed and wheelchair wheels are locked to prevent movement during ambulation; ensure the patient is wearing rubber-soled socks or shoes to prevent slipping; and make sure the patient is not suffering from any dizziness or lightheadedness that may result from a quick change in position. Lift the leg pads and footplates up and out of the way to prevent tripping. Explain the procedure to the patient. Assist the patient into a dangling position. Place your feet in a wide stance. Instruct the patient to stand on the count of three, and support the torso while helping the patient into a standing position. Pivot the patient so that his back is to the wheelchair. Instruct the patient to position his arms on the armrests of the wheelchair and back up until he feels the seat against the backs of his legs. Slowly lower the patient into a sitting position. Assist the patient in lifting his legs and placing the leg pads and footplates beneath them.

Transferring a patient to side of the bed

Patient strength should be assessed prior to moving the patient to determine how much assistance may be required. While the patient is in bed, make sure the brakes are locked and the bed is in the lowest position. Lower the side rail, and raise the head of the bed until it is at a comfortable level for the patient. While facing the patient, place one arm behind the shoulders and one arm beneath the knees. Assist the patient into a sitting position at the side of the bed. Allow the patient to remain there for a few moments to ensure the patient is not dizzy from the change in position.

Transferring the patient from bed to stretcher

While the patient is lying in bed, make sure the wheels of the bed and the stretcher are locked. Raise the level of the bed until it is the same height as the stretcher. If available, a slider board can be placed beneath the patient to facilitate movement and decrease friction. Stand at the side of the stretcher, and ask a colleague to stand next to the bed. Instruct the patient to cross his arms over his chest to prevent dragging his limbs across the bed. Grasp the draw sheet, and roll it to maintain a good grip. On the count of three, pull the draw sheet toward you, while the colleague at the side of the bed pushes the patient from the other side. Continue to pull until the patient is in the center of the stretcher. Position the patient for comfort.

SBA, CGA, MIN, and MAX

Stand By Assistance (SBA), Contact Guard Assistance (CGA), Minimum (MIN), and Maximum (MAX) assistance refer to the level of assistance the patient requires while ambulating. A patient who can move independently requires SBA. This patient does not require any assistance in ambulating and does not require a gait belt. CGA refers to a patient who does not require assistance but is at risk for falling. The patient care technician should be close enough to touch the patient in case he should fall, but does not provide additional support. MIN assistance refers to the patient who needs a small amount of support while ambulating. A gait belt is advised for this type of patient. Patients who require MAX assistance may or may not be able to bear their own weight. This type of patient requires support from one or two staff members to ensure that he does not fall.

Crutches

Ambulation
The swing-to and swing-through methods of crutch walking are intended for patients who have decreased lower body strength. Both methods are advantageous in that they are easy to learn and allow for a quick gait. The disadvantage is that both methods require strong upper body strength. In the swing-to method, both crutches are moved forward and placed at the length of a step in front of them. The patient then places his weight upon the crutches and swings his body forward until his feet are equal to the crutches. In the swing-through method, both crutches are moved forward. Placing his weight upon the crutches, the patient swings his lower body forward and places his feet slightly in front of the crutches.

The four-point technique is the preferred method of ambulation for a patient with poor lower body strength who is ambulating with crutches. While the patient is standing, instruct him to move the left crutch forward first, followed by the right foot. The right crutch should then be moved forward, followed by the left foot. The advantage of this method of ambulation is that the patient has at least three points of contact with the ground at all times, offering the most stability; the disadvantage is that it requires a slow movement speed. The three-point technique is recommended for patients who are unable to bear weight on one foot while ambulating with crutches. While in a standing position, the patient should move both crutches and the affected limb forward. Then, while placing his weight on the crutches, the patient should move his strong leg forward until it is even with the affected extremity.

<u>Transferring a patient from sitting to standing</u>
While the patient is sitting in the chair, instruct him to hold both crutches in one hand by gripping the handgrips. Instruct the patient to scoot his hips to the edge of the chair and stretch the non-weight-bearing foot out straight. Help the patient rise to a standing position, using the arm of the chair to support one of the patient's arms and the crutches to support the other. Once the patient has balanced his weight on one foot, instruct the patient to move one of the crutches to the opposite side and place his hands on the handgrips.

Transferring a patient from standing to sitting

To move from a standing to a sitting position, instruct the patient to approach the chair until he is one step away from the front of the chair. Instruct the patient to carefully turn using his weight-bearing leg and the crutches until his back is to the chair. Assist the patient in finding his balance before transferring one of the crutches to the opposite side. Instruct the patient to grip both crutches by the handgrips. Help the patient to reach back with his free hand to find the arm of the chair. Instruct the patient to stretch the non-weight-bearing foot in front of him. Assist the patient with slowly lowering his weight into the chair.

<u>Fit</u>
Though it is the job of the physical therapist to adjust crutches properly to the size of the patient, the crutch should be checked prior to each ambulation to make sure it continues to fit properly. The pads of the crutch should remain one to one-and-a-half inches below the axillary area. The handgrips should be even with the patient's hips. When the patient is in a standing position with hands resting on the handgrips, his elbows should be slightly flexed. When the patient walks on crutches, he should support his weight with his hands on the handgrips. Placing his weight on the pads in the axillary area may cause nerve damage. The patient should keep the head and shoulders erect to limit back strain and keep the torso aligned with the crutches to prevent loss of balance and injury.

Ambulating a patient with a walker

A patient, who is learning to ambulate with a walker, should wear a gait belt at all times. Instruct the patient to stand in the middle of the walker, holding it by the handgrips. Instruct the patient to move the walker forward until the back legs are even with the toes. While keeping his weight on the strong leg, the patient should then take a step forward with the weaker leg, until it is in the center of the walker. Then, instruct the patient to place his weight upon the handgrips while taking a step forward with his strong leg. Once he has regained his balance, repeat the process.

Sitting position to standing with a walker

While the patient is sitting in the chair, open the walker and place it in front of him. Make sure the patient is wearing a gait belt. Instruct the patient to scoot forward until he is sitting on the edge of the chair. Instruct the patient to place both hands on the arms of the chair. On the count of three, assist the patient into a standing position. While providing support for the patient, instruct him to move his hands, one at a time, from the arms of the chair to the handgrips of the walker. Wait a moment to ensure the patient is not dizzy before beginning to ambulate.

Ambulating a patient with a cane

While ambulating a patient who is learning how to walk with a cane, always provide the patient with a gait belt. Instruct the patient to hold the cane in his strong hand. As the patient takes a step forward with the affected extremity, advance the cane forward, keeping the cane even with the leg and the patient's full weight upon his strong leg. Once the weakened leg and the cane are in place, instruct the patient to place his weight upon the cane while taking a step forward with the unaffected extremity. Allow the patient a moment to regain his balance before repeating the process.

Safety during ambulation

While the patient is ambulating, make sure to provide support using a gait belt. Ensure the patient is wearing rubber-soled slippers. If the patient is receiving oxygen therapy, obtain a rolling tank so the patient can continue to wear oxygen while ambulating. Carefully monitor the patient's respirations, and frequently check to make sure the patient is not becoming fatigued or dizzy. Move at a pace that is comfortable for the patient, and do not try to rush him. If necessary, allow the patient to stop to take a brief rest in a chair to ensure that he does not become overexerted.

Moving the patient up in the bed

Never try to move a patient up in bed by yourself. Always ask another patient care technician or nurse to help you. Prior to moving the patient up in bed, explain to the patient what you are going to do. Wash your hands, and don a pair of gloves. Lay the head of the bed as flat as possible, and raise the level of the bed until it is a comfortable height for you. Position yourself near the head of the bed on one side, while the other person moves to the opposite side of the bed. Instruct the patient to cross his arms over his chest to prevent his limbs from dragging and to tuck his chin to his chest. If the patient is unable to do so, support the back of his neck with one hand. Grasp the draw sheet and roll the edge to establish a good grip. On the count of three, lift the draw sheet and pull upward. Position the patient for comfort.

Placing the patient in a side-lying position

Wash your hands, don a pair of gloves, and explain to the patient what you are going to do. Obtain assistance to help turn the patient. Raise the level of the bed to a comfortable height. Using the draw sheet, move the patient closer to the side of the bed opposite of the direction you intend to turn him; this will allow the patient to remain in the center of the bed after having been turned. Grasp the draw sheet and use it to pull the patient onto his side. If the patient is able, ask him to grasp the side rail while you position him. Tuck a pillow beneath the patient's back, under the draw sheet. Tuck another pillow beneath the patient's buttocks. Place a pillow underneath the patient's arm and between the patient's knees for support. Remove your gloves, and wash your hands.

Supine, prone, Sims', lateral, semi-Fowler's, and high-Fowler's positions

When the patient is in a supine position, he is lying flat on the back, with arms extended at the sides. A prone position consists of the patient resting on the stomach, with the head turned to one side on the pillow and arms extended at the side. When the patient is in the

Sims' position, he should be positioned on his side, with both legs straight. The lateral position is similar to the Sims' position in that the patient is lying on the side. However, in the lateral position, the patient's topmost leg is flexed. Both the flexed leg and topmost arm are elevated on a pillow for additional support. The semi-Fowler's position consists of the patient lying on the back with the head of the bed at a 45-degree angle. A high-Fowler's position is similar to the semi-Fowler's, however, the head of the bed is raised to a 90-degree angle.

Logrolling a patient

Logrolling is a procedure that is performed whenever the patient has sustained a neck or spinal cord injury. Ideally, patients with this type of injury should be turned as little as possible until the neck or spine has been stabilized. In certain cases, turning cannot be avoided, such as if the patient has become incontinent. If the patient must be moved, the head, neck, and back must be kept in a stable position to prevent further injury. This requires good communication among the caregivers who are moving the patient to ensure that their movements are coordinated to maintain proper alignment.

Logrolling a patient requires a minimum of three people in order to be performed successfully. Wash your hands, don a pair of gloves, and explain what you are going to do. Have one person positioned at the patient's head, and two others on the side in which the patient is to be facing. Grasp the draw sheet, and turn the patient. The person at the head of the bed should keep the patient's head midline with the rest of the body, while the people at the side of the bed keep the back and hips in alignment. Perform the necessary procedures, and then return the patient to his back. It is imperative that the patient's head, neck, and back are kept in alignment. Position the patient for comfort, and wash your hands.

Practice Test

Practice Questions

1. What is the term used to described the ventricular volume at the end of diastole?
    a. Preload
    b. Stroke volume
    c. Afterload
    d. End-systolic volume

2. What does the term edema mean?
    a. Rash
    b. Within
    c. Vomiting
    d. Swelling

3. If a patient is lying on their back, they are in a _____ position.
    a. Prone
    b. Prostrate
    c. Dorsal
    d. Supine

4. What does the prefix dys- mean?
    a. Discharge
    b. Around
    c. Difficult
    d. After

5. Which of the following definitions match the term neurasthenia?
    a. inflammation of a nerve
    b. nerve weakness
    c. condition of a nerve
    d. abnormal nerve protrusion

6. Which of the following definitions match the term osteoblast?
    a. condition of the ear
    b. bone developing cell
    c. pertaining to bone destruction
    d. an intervertebral condition

7. Which of the following definitions match the term carpectomy?
    a. excision of cartilage from a joint
    b. excision of cartilage from the neck
    c. excision of bone from the hand
    d. excision of bone from the foot

8. Which of the following definitions match the term patellectomy?
    a. incision made in the patella
    b. pertaining to the patella
    c. fusion of the patella
    d. removal of the patella

9. HIPAA guarantees a patient's right to:
    a. confidentiality.
    b. informed consent.
    c. see their chart.
    d. continuity of care.

10. A patient has a few questions about the consent forms she signed for a scheduled invasive procedure. How should the Patient Care Technician respond?
    a. Answer the questions to the best of her ability.
    b. Tell the patient that she will ask the nurse to contact the doctor.
    c. Tell the patient that she will have plenty of time to ask the doctor before the procedure.
    d. Remind the patient that she signed the consent and that the procedure has already been scheduled.

11. Which heart chamber functions to pump deoxygenated blood to the lungs?
    a. Right atrium
    b. Right ventricle
    c. Left atrium
    d. Left ventricle

12. Which lead is the most affected by respiration?
    a. V2
    b. V4
    c. Lead III
    d. Lead I

13. Which of the following is the correct sequence by which action potentials are conducted through the heart?
    a. SA node → AV node → bundle branches → Purkinje fibers
    b. Bundle branches → Purkinje fibers → SA node → AV node
    c. Purkinje fibers → SA node → bundle branches → AV node
    d. AV node → SA node → bundle branches → Purkinje fibers

14. What type of heart block is seen in the following electrocardiogram (ECG) strip?

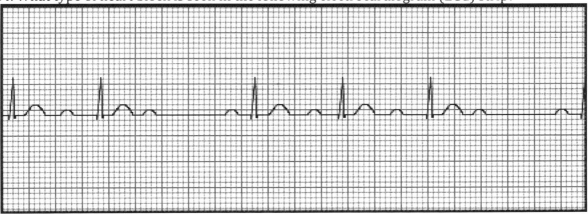

    a. First-degree heart block
    b. Second-degree heart block, type 1
    c. Second-degree heart block, type 2
    d. Third-degree heart block

15. When calibrating an ECG machine, what is the standard size of the calibration mark representing the sensitivity of the ECG machine?
    a. 5 mm in height
    b. 10 mm in height
    c. 15 mm in height
    d. 20 mm in height

16. How many leaflets does the mitral valve have?
    a. One
    b. Two
    c. Three
    d. Four

17. The right and left coronary arteries branch off of which blood vessel?
    a. Ascending aorta
    b. Descending aorta
    c. Pulmonary artery
    d. Posterior descending artery

18. How are cardiac cells able to depolarize spontaneously and thus demonstrate automaticity?
    a. They are consistently triggered by the sympathetic nervous system
    b. They have an unstable resting potential that allows influx of calcium and sodium
    c. They have increased permeability to potassium ions while in a resting state
    d. Parasympathetic nervous system fibers regularly trigger the cells

19. A patient is anxious and begins hyperventilating. His hands and lips start to feel numb and tingly, and he feels lightheaded. What is the physiological cause of his symptoms?
    a. Excess carbon dioxide in the blood
    b. Excess oxygen in the blood
    c. Lack of carbon dioxide in the blood
    d. Lack of oxygen in the blood

20. When food is traveling through the gastrointestinal system, what part of the small intestine does it enter immediately after leaving the stomach?
    a. Jejunum
    b. Duodenum
    c. Ileum
    d. Rectum

21. A patient comes into the clinic complaining of weight loss, anxiety, sweating, and diarrhea. She is diagnosed with hyperthyroidism. The thyroid gland is part of what body system?
    a. Nervous system
    b. Musculoskeletal system
    c. Digestive system
    d. Endocrine system

22. Which of the following is obesity LEAST likely to play a role in?
    a. Osteoporosis
    b. Gallstones
    c. Osteoarthritis
    d. Type II diabetes

23. Glucagon increases blood levels of glucose by causing liver to breakdown glycogen.
    a. TRUE
    b. FALSE

24. Which of the following is not an indicator of a hypoglycemic condition?
    a. Fatigue
    b. Poor appetite
    c. Tachycardia
    d. Confusion

25. What type of cells secrete insulin?
    a. Beta cells
    b. Alpha cells
    c. Plasma cells
    d. Acinar cells

26. What type of cell releases glucagon?
    a. β cells
    b. α cells
    c. plasma cells
    d. Δ cells

27. Which of the following is the outermost layer of the epidermis?
    a. Stratum spinosum
    b. Stratum corneum
    c. Stratum granulosum
    d. Stratum basale

28. The innermost layer of a blood vessel is lined with _____ _____ cells
    a. Simple squamous
    b. Stratified squamous
    c. Simple cuboidal epithelium
    d. Stratified cuboidal epithelium

29. Which of the following is the standard respiration rate for adults?
    a. 10-20 breaths/min.
    b. 12-20 breaths/min.
    c. 8-15 breaths/min.
    d. 12-18 breaths/min.

30. Which of the following items requires cleaning with a disinfectant prior to use?
    a. Stethoscope
    b. Scalpel
    c. Thermometer
    d. Blood pressure cuff

31. What is the proper term for an infection that is transmitted during a medical procedure?
    a. Droplet
    b. Iatrogenic
    c. Direct oral contact
    d. Fecal-oral transmission

32. Which of the following is NOT required to be on the label of a medical specimen?
    a. Date of collection
    b. Time of collection
    c. The patient's full name
    d. Full name and signature of the person collecting the specimen

33. What instructions should be given to a female patient when a clean-catch urine sample is needed?
    a. Use a sterile wipe to clean between the labial folds, wiping from back to front.
    b. Include the initial stream of urine in the sample.
    c. Do not allow the labial folds to become spread open.
    d. Urinate a small amount into the toilet bowl, then collect the sample using the urine cup.

34. Which of the following is an appropriate site for an intramuscular injection?
    a. Triceps muscle
    b. Dorsogluteal muscle
    c. Quadriceps femoris muscle
    d. Soleus muscle

35. Which of the following actions does NOT help prevent the contamination of blood samples?
   a. Wiping the shaft of the needle used to draw the blood sample with an alcohol swab
   b. Disinfecting the patient's skin in the area the blood is to be drawn
   c. Washing your hands before drawing the blood sample
   d. Wearing gloves

36. A yellow cap on a tube stopper indicates the presence of which additive?
   a. Sodium citrate
   b. Sodium fluoride
   c. SPS
   d. EDTA

37. When performing a bed bath, what temperature should the water be?
   a. 70-80 degrees Fahrenheit
   b. 105-115 degrees Fahrenheit
   c. 130-140 degrees Fahrenheit
   d. 155-165 degrees Fahrenheit

38. How would you classify a pressure sore that has a pink wound bed, but does not extend through the full thickness of the skin?
   a. Stage I
   b. Stage II
   c. Stage III
   d. Stage IV

39. A patient is scheduled for surgery later in the day. What type of food would you expect on his breakfast tray?
   a. No tray – the patient is NPO
   b. Jell-O and chicken broth
   c. Scrambled eggs
   d. French toast and fruit

40. For a patient on fall precautions, what is the minimum number of side rails that should be raised while the patient is in bed?
   a. 1
   b. 2
   c. 3
   d. 4

41. Which technique is MOST appropriate for a patient with both poor upper body and lower body strength?
   a. Four-point technique
   b. Three-point technique
   c. Swing-to method
   d. Swing-through method

42. There is a note on a patient's chart that she should be placed in the Sim's position. How should the patient be positioned?
     a. Lying on the stomach with the head turned to the side
     b. On her back with the head of the bed raised to a 90 degree angle
     c. On her back with the head of the bed raised to a 45 degree angle
     d. On her left side with the top leg flexed and supported by a pillow

43. When caring for a patient with diarrhea, which of the following should be recorded in the patient's chart?
     a. Odor of the stool
     b. Types and amounts of fluids the patient is drinking
     c. Number of stools
     d. All of the above

44. What is one technique a Patient Care Technician can use to help a patient with aphasia?
     a. Providing a time limit for the patient to respond
     b. Speaking for the patient
     c. Using a picture or letter board
     d. Giving the patient a pen

45. Which of the following answer choices correctly lists the five stages of grief in order of their expected occurrence?
     a. Denial, anger, bargaining, depression, acceptance
     b. Anger, denial, depression, bargaining, acceptance
     c. Depression, denial, anger, bargaining, acceptance
     d. Bargaining, denial, anger, depression, acceptance

46. When the Patient Care Technician is informed of an admission, what is her responsibility?
     a. Prepare the room, including the linens, gowns, and other necessary equipment.
     b. Complete the admissions interview.
     c. Make sure the patient's medications have been received from the pharmacy and are correct.
     d. Coordinate the patient's care with the rest of the treatment team.

47. What is the appropriate way to take a radial pulse?
     a. Place your index finger and middle finger on the wrist, under the pinky finger.
     b. Place your index finger and middle finger on the wrist, under the thumb.
     c. Place your thumb on the side of the neck, next to the trachea.
     d. Place your index finger on the inner side of the upper arm, about halfway between the shoulder and the elbow.

48. A six-month-old baby in the waiting room suddenly begins to choke on a small toy. The baby's mother yells for help. You run into the room to assist and see that the baby is still conscious, but she is unable to cough or make crying noises. What steps should you take to try to relieve the obstruction?

a. Lay the infant on the ground and give quick, consecutive thrusts on the middle of the breastbone with two fingers. After every 30 compressions, try to visualize the object that is blocking the airway.

b. Open the baby's mouth and sweep your finger into the back of her throat to try to dislodge the obstructing object.

c. Lay the infant face-down along your arm, cradling her jaw in your fingers. Using the palm of your other hand, give the baby five quick, firm blows on the back between the shoulder blades. Then, turn the infant face-up and give five quick thrusts on the middle of the breastbone with two fingers.

d. Hold the infant on your lap, facing away from you. Use your fist to forcefully press inward and upward just under the breastbone.

49. Which of the following locations will yield the most accurate results when taking an infant's temperature?

a. Mouth
b. Armpit
c. Rectum
d. Ear

50. What information should be recorded on all patient visit notes?

a. Time and date
b. Patient signature
c. Patient Social Security number
d. Physician's provider number

Answers and Explanations

1. A: The ventricular volume at the end of diastole is the preload. Stroke volume is the amount of blood that is pumped from the left ventricle in one contraction. Afterload is the end load against which the heart must overcome to eject blood. End-systolic volume is the ventricular volume after contraction.

3. D: The term edema means swelling. The swelling is caused by an accumulation of fluid within the tissues of the body. Exanthema refers to a rash. The prefix endo- means within. The suffix -emesis refers to vomiting.

3. D: The definition of supine is lying on the back with the face upward or having the palm of the hand facing upward. Prone is the position of lying on the stomach or having the palm of the hand facing downward. Dorsal refers to the back of the body. Prostrate is defined as being stretched out, face-down.

4. C: The prefix dys- means abnormal or difficult. Examples include dysphagia, which means difficulty swallowing, and dysplasia, which means the abnormal growth of tissues or cells. The suffix -rrhea means discharge. The prefix peri- means around. The prefix post- means after.

5. B: Nerve weakness

6. B: Bone developing cell

7. C: Excision of bone from the hand

8. D: Removal of the patella

9. A: HIPAA guarantees a patient's confidentiality and privacy. It also requires healthcare providers to provide patients with a list of policies that have been designed to protect their privacy. Only providers who are directly caring for someone should have access to their medical chart.

10. B: A Patient Care Technician should not discuss procedures or what was in the consent forms the patient signed. Only a physician can review and inform a patient of the risks and benefits of having a procedure or treatment. A patient can always withdraw their consent, even if they're about to go into the procedure room. The nurse should notify the physician that the patient has questions so he can arrange to see the patient and discuss her concerns.

11. B: The right ventricle pumps the deoxygenated blood it has received from the right atrium to the lungs. The right atrium pumps deoxygenated blood from the body to the right ventricle. The left atrium pumps oxygenated blood from the lungs to the left ventricle. The left ventricle pumps oxygenated blood to the body.

12. C: Lead III is the most affected by respiration, and therefore the waveforms may look different depending on the respiratory cycle. Because of this, a Q wave that *only* appears in lead III and is not associated with other corresponding changes in other leads is not significant.

13. A: The sequence by which an action potential is conducted through the heart is from the sinoatrial (SA) node to the atrioventricular (AV) node to the bundle branches and then to the Purkinje fibers.

14. B: The pictured ECG is a second-degree heart block, type 1. This rhythm is also called Mobitz I or Wenckebach. With this heart block the PR interval gets longer with each beat until eventually a P wave occurs, but a QRS does not follow (a beat is skipped). After the skipped beat, the pattern starts over again. A first-degree heart block occurs when the PR interval is longer than 0.2 seconds, but the PR interval generally remains constant and the QRS is not dropped. A second-degree heart block, type 2, also called Mobitz II, is apparent when the QRS suddenly fails to show up after a P wave. A fairly consistent ratio of P waves to QRS complexes is common, and this rhythm lacks the increasing PR interval that is seen in the Mobitz I block. A third-degree heart block is also called a complete heart block and the atria and ventricles beat independently of one another.

15. B: The calibration mark representing the sensitivity of the ECG should be 10 mm in height (two large squares). This mark is usually found on the left side of the page at the beginning of each line of the ECG. When this is set correctly it means that for every millivolt measured from the patient, a deflection of 10 mm will be recorded on the trace.

16. B: The mitral valve is a bicuspid valve, meaning that it has two leaflets (also known as cusps). It is located between the left atrium and left ventricle. The tricuspid valve, located between the right atrium and right ventricle, has three leaflets. The pulmonic valve leads from the right ventricle to the pulmonary artery and has three leaflets. The aortic valve leads from the left ventricle to the aorta and normally has three leaflets.

17. A: The right and left coronary arteries branch off from the root of the ascending aorta. The root of the ascending aorta refers to the beginning of the aorta, immediately after it exits the left ventricle.

18. B: Certain cardiac cells spontaneously depolarize, which is referred to as automaticity. The depolarization of the cell leads to an action potential being formed. Spontaneously depolarizing cardiac cells, such as those in the SA node, have unstable resting potentials created by positive sodium and calcium ions flowing slowly and continuously into the cell while the cell is at rest. As a result of the inflow of positive ions, the cell slowly depolarizes until it reaches a point where it triggers a change in membrane permeability. This change allows for the positively charged ions (mainly sodium) to move more quickly into the cell, depolarizing it further until an action potential is produced. The plasma membranes of these cells have reduced permeability to potassium while at rest. The sympathetic and parasympathetic nervous systems can change the heart rate, but this is not considered "spontaneous" or "automaticity."

19. C: Hyperventilation refers to a patient breathing more quickly than normal. This rapid rate of ventilation results in carbon dioxide being exhaled at a higher rate than normal. This can result in metabolic alkalosis, meaning that the pH of the blood is abnormally elevated. The symptoms that may accompany hyperventilation are related to the metabolic alkalosis that develops. The patient should be reassured in a calm manner to reduce anxiety. Have the patient sit down and instruct him to take slow, deep breaths.

20. B: The small intestine is divided into three major parts. The duodenum is the first section, just distal to the stomach; the jejunum is the middle section; and the ileum is the third section that connects to the large intestine.

21. D: The endocrine system consists of a group of glands that secretes hormones into the blood. These hormones play important roles in regulating various functions of the body. With hyperthyroidism, there is excess thyroid hormone being secreted by the thyroid gland, and this can cause a number of symptoms, including weight loss, anxiety, sweating, and diarrhea.

22. A: Obesity is associated with numerous health problems. These include gallstones, osteoarthritis, type II diabetes, heart disease, hypertension, and various types of cancer. It was previously thought that obese patients were LESS likely to have osteoporosis than nonobese patients, but new research is questioning this theory. Obesity has been directly linked to the other listed health problems, but research is still ongoing about the association between obesity and osteoporosis.

23. A: True

24. B: Poor appetite

25. A: Beta cells

26. B: α cells

27. B: Stratum corneum

28. A: Simple squamous

29. B: 12-20 breaths/min.

30. C: Items that require cleaning with a disinfectant are ones that come into contact with a patient's mucus membranes but don't puncture the skin. Thermometers and respiratory equipment are good examples of items that should be disinfected but don't require sterilization. Items such as scalpels that penetrate the skin should be sterilized between patients because of the high risk of contamination. Items such as stethoscopes and blood pressure cuffs that just touch the skin can be cleaned with a mild detergent between uses.

31. B: An infection that is transmitted during a medical procedure is called iatrogenic. Droplet transmission is when bacteria or viruses are released in droplets when a person sneezes or coughs. Direct oral contact is transmission between people when there is direct oral contact, such as kissing or sharing a drinking cup. Fecal-oral contamination is exactly what it sounds like: fecal material contaminates food, usually through poor hand washing or poor food preparation techniques.

32. D: When labeling medical specimens (e.g., blood, urine, or sputum) it is important to include the date and time of collection, the type of specimen, and the patient's full name and date of birth or medical record number. Although the full name and signature of the person

collecting the specimen are not required, the collector should include his or her initials on the label.

33. D: When a clean-catch urine sample is needed from a female patient, she should be instructed to sit on the toilet, spread open the labial folds with two fingers, use a sterile wipe to clean the inner folds of the labia (wiping from front to back), and use a second wipe to clean the area over the urethra. The patient should then urinate a small amount into the toilet bowl, temporarily stop the flow of urine, and then collect a urine sample using the urine cup.

34. B: The four sites most appropriate for intramuscular injections are the deltoid muscle, the vastus lateralis muscle, the ventrogluteal muscle, and the dorsogluteal muscle. The deltoid muscle is located in the upper arm. The vastus lateralis muscle is located in the thigh. The ventrogluteal muscle is located in the hip. The dorsogluteal muscle is the large muscle in the buttock. When selecting which site to use, you should consider the age of the patient, the medication that is being injected, and the general condition of the patient.

35. A: The needles used for blood collection come in sterile packaging. After uncapping the needle, it is best to avoid touching its shaft (the part of the needle that will puncture the patient's skin). Wiping the needle with an alcohol swab is unnecessary because the needle is already sterile. Disinfecting the patient's skin, washing your hands, and wearing gloves will all help prevent contamination of blood samples.

36. C: SPS

37. B: Water for a bed bath should be heated up to approximately 105 to 115 degrees Fahrenheit. Any cooler and the water will cool off too much before the end of the bath, chilling the patient. Any warmer and the water will be too hot, and could potentially burn the patient. Filling the basin should be the last thing you do; gather all other supplies first to minimize the cooling of the water. If you don't have a thermometer to measure the water temperature, make sure it is comfortably warm against your elbow or inner arm.

38. B: A stage I pressure sore would appear as a reddened area that does not blanch (turn white) when pressed. A stage II pressure sore involves a partial breakdown of the upper layer of skin, but does not extend all the way through the skin. A stage II pressure ulcer may look like a blister. Stage III and stage IV ulcers extend all the way through the skin. You may see the underlying subcutaneous fat in a stage III ulcer, whereas a stage IV may proceed all the way down to the muscles, tendons, or bones. Make sure to report any skin redness to the nurse so that the skin can be thoroughly assessed.

39. A: A patient who is about to undergo surgery or another procedure requiring an anesthetic should be NPO for a minimum of eight hours before the procedure. If the patient receives a tray, you should double check with the nurse before serving the patient his breakfast. If a procedure is scheduled for later in the day, the anesthesiologist may be okay with the patient eating breakfast.

40. B: A minimum of two bed rails should be raised when the patient is in bed. Raising four side rails is considered a restraint, and should not be done unless directly ordered by the physician. One raised bed rail leaves an entire side of the bed without any boundaries.

41. A: Four-point technique is a great method of crutch walking for patients who have poor upper and lower body strength because it balances out the patient's weight on both arms and the alternating legs. Three-point, swing-to, and swing-through methods are all great for a patient who has good upper body strength because these gaits depend primarily on the arms to keep the patient upright.

42. D: Sim's position is when a patient is lying on her side with the top leg flexed towards the chest. Choice A, on her stomach, is called the prone position. Choice B, with the head of the bed raised to a 90 degree angle, is called the High Fowler's position. Choice C, on her back with the head of the bed raised to 45 degrees, is called the Semi-Fowler's position.

43. D: When caring for a patient with diarrhea, it is important to note all of the information in the answer choices in the patient's chart, as it can be vitally important to the care and treatment plan for the patient. Additionally, the doctor will need the information to gauge the severity of the diarrhea and dehydration. The Patient Care Technician should also note how much fluid is passed with each stool and how often the patient is having episodes of diarrhea.

44. C: Aphasia is an acquired inability to understand language and express oneself through speech. Patients with aphasia have different levels of ability, and should be approached with patience. Setting a time limit and speaking for the patient are not productive or helpful in terms of helping the patient relearn these skills. A pen and paper may be helpful in some situations, but many patients aren't able to read or write as a result of their aphasia. A picture or letter board is a universal method of communication, and offers an easy way to communicate because it is so simple to use.

45. A: The first stage of grief is denial that the event happened or is going to happen. Following that is anger at the situation or people involved. Next is bargaining, in which the sufferer bargains with God (I'll do…… if you make this go away). Depression follows as the person starts to deal with their grief. Finally, the patient begins to accept what has happened and can start to move forward. It's important to keep in mind that not everyone goes through the same steps in a linear and straightforward manner. It's not uncommon for someone to progress through one stage quickly and then get held up at a subsequent stage or even regress back to a prior stage.

46. A: The Patient Care Technician should prepare the room, ensuring that linens, personal protective equipment, and other medical supplies are present. The Patient Care Technician should also help orient the patient to the unit and take vital signs. The nurse should complete the admission interview and assessment and coordinate all aspects of care. This includes contacting the pharmacy and ensuring the correct medications are received.

47. B: The radial pulse is palpated at the wrist, under the thumb. When taking a pulse, you should use the pads of your index finger and middle finger. Your thumb has a pulse beat of its own, which may interfere with feeling the patient's pulse. The carotid pulse is palpated on the side of the neck, next to the trachea. The brachial pulse is palpated on the inner side of the upper arm, about halfway between the shoulder and elbow. The ulnar artery pulse is located at the wrist, under the pinky, but it is not as commonly used as the radial pulse.

48. C: Answer C describes the correct way to provide choking first aid to a conscious child under the age of one. You continue to repeat the five back blows and five chest thrusts until

- 133 -

the object is dislodged or until the baby becomes unconscious. Answer A describes infant CPR, which is what should be done if the choking baby becomes unconscious. You should not perform blind finger sweeps, as described in B because this may push the object further into the throat. If you can visualize the object, you can try to reach in and pull it out. Answer D describes how you would do the Heimlich maneuver in an older child or adult.

49. C: A rectal temperature reading is considered the most accurate for infants. Other methods can be used to take an infant's temperature, but it is important to get the most accurate reading as possible in infants because their health is generally more delicate than that of older children. The closer the thermometer is to the inside of the body, the warmer and more accurate the temperature will be.

50. A: The correct time and date should be recorded on all patient documents. In addition, often the patient's name, birth date, and medical record number are included on documents. There are several types of documents that do require the patient's signature, Social Security number, and other personal information, but this information is not required on *all* patient visit documentation. The physician's provider number is used for health insurance purposes, and it is not required to be written on all patient visit notes.

Secret Key #1 - Time is Your Greatest Enemy

Pace Yourself

Wear a watch. At the beginning of the test, check the time (or start a chronometer on your watch to count the minutes), and check the time after every few questions to make sure you are "on schedule."

If you are forced to speed up, do it efficiently. Usually one or more answer choices can be eliminated without too much difficulty. Above all, don't panic. Don't speed up and just begin guessing at random choices. By pacing yourself, and continually monitoring your progress against your watch, you will always know exactly how far ahead or behind you are with your available time. If you find that you are one minute behind on the test, don't skip one question without spending any time on it, just to catch back up. Take 15 fewer seconds on the next four questions, and after four questions you'll have caught back up. Once you catch back up, you can continue working each problem at your normal pace.

Furthermore, don't dwell on the problems that you were rushed on. If a problem was taking up too much time and you made a hurried guess, it must be difficult. The difficult questions are the ones you are most likely to miss anyway, so it isn't a big loss. It is better to end with more time than you need than to run out of time.

Lastly, sometimes it is beneficial to slow down if you are constantly getting ahead of time. You are always more likely to catch a careless mistake by working more slowly than quickly, and among very high-scoring test takers (those who are likely to have lots of time left over), careless errors affect the score more than mastery of material.

Secret Key #2 - Guessing is not Guesswork

You probably know that guessing is a good idea. Unlike other standardized tests, there is no penalty for getting a wrong answer. Even if you have no idea about a question, you still have a 20-25% chance of getting it right.

Most test takers do not understand the impact that proper guessing can have on their score. Unless you score extremely high, guessing will significantly contribute to your final score.

Monkeys Take the Test

What most test takers don't realize is that to insure that 20-25% chance, you have to guess randomly. If you put 20 monkeys in a room to take this test, assuming they answered once per question and behaved themselves, on average they would get 20-25% of the questions correct. Put 20 test takers in the room, and the average will be much lower among guessed questions. Why?

    1. The test writers intentionally write deceptive answer choices that "look" right. A test

- 135 -

taker has no idea about a question, so he picks the "best looking" answer, which is often wrong. The monkey has no idea what looks good and what doesn't, so it will consistently be right about 20-25% of the time.

2. Test takers will eliminate answer choices from the guessing pool based on a hunch or intuition. Simple but correct answers often get excluded, leaving a 0% chance of being correct. The monkey has no clue, and often gets lucky with the best choice.

This is why the process of elimination endorsed by most test courses is flawed and detrimental to your performance. Test takers don't guess; they make an ignorant stab in the dark that is usually worse than random.

$5 Challenge

Let me introduce one of the most valuable ideas of this course—the $5 challenge:

You only mark your "best guess" if you are willing to bet $5 on it.
You only eliminate choices from guessing if you are willing to bet $5 on it.

Why $5? Five dollars is an amount of money that is small yet not insignificant, and can really add up fast (20 questions could cost you $100). Likewise, each answer choice on one question of the test will have a small impact on your overall score, but it can really add up to a lot of points in the end.

The process of elimination IS valuable. The following shows your chance of guessing it right:

If you eliminate wrong answer choices until only this many remain:	Chance of getting it correct:
1	100%
2	50%
3	33%

However, if you accidentally eliminate the right answer or go on a hunch for an incorrect answer, your chances drop dramatically—to 0%. By guessing among all the answer choices, you are GUARANTEED to have a shot at the right answer.

That's why the $5 test is so valuable. If you give up the advantage and safety of a pure guess, it had better be worth the risk.

What we still haven't covered is how to be sure that whatever guess you make is truly random. Here's the easiest way:

Always pick the first answer choice among those remaining.

Such a technique means that you have decided, **before you see a single test question**, exactly how you are going to guess, and since the order of choices tells you nothing about which one is correct, this guessing technique is perfectly random.

This section is not meant to scare you away from making educated guesses or eliminating choices; you just need to define when a choice is worth eliminating. The $5 test, along with a pre-defined random guessing strategy, is the best way to make sure you reap all of the benefits of guessing.

Secret Key #3 - Practice Smarter, Not Harder

Many test takers delay the test preparation process because they dread the awful amounts of practice time they think necessary to succeed on the test. We have refined an effective method that will take you only a fraction of the time.

There are a number of "obstacles" in the path to success. Among these are answering questions, finishing in time, and mastering test-taking strategies. All must be executed on the day of the test at peak performance, or your score will suffer. The test is a mental marathon that has a large impact on your future.

Just like a marathon runner, it is important to work your way up to the full challenge. So first you just worry about questions, and then time, and finally strategy:

Success Strategy

1. Find a good source for practice tests.
2. If you are willing to make a larger time investment, consider using more than one study guide. Often the different approaches of multiple authors will help you "get" difficult concepts.
3. Take a practice test with no time constraints, with all study helps, "open book." Take your time with questions and focus on applying strategies.
4. Take a practice test with time constraints, with all guides, "open book."
5. Take a final practice test without open material and with time limits.

If you have time to take more practice tests, just repeat step 5. By gradually exposing yourself to the full rigors of the test environment, you will condition your mind to the stress of test day and maximize your success.

Secret Key #4 - Prepare, Don't Procrastinate

Let me state an obvious fact: if you take the test three times, you will probably get three different scores. This is due to the way you feel on test day, the level of preparedness you have, and the version of the test you see. Despite the test writers' claims to the contrary, some versions of the test WILL be easier for you than others.

Since your future depends so much on your score, you should maximize your chances of success. In order to maximize the likelihood of success, you've got to prepare in advance. This means taking practice tests and spending time learning the information and test taking strategies you will need to succeed.

Never go take the actual test as a "practice" test, expecting that you can just take it again if you need to. Take all the practice tests you can on your own, but when you go to take the official test, be prepared, be focused, and do your best the first time!

Secret Key #5 - Test Yourself

Everyone knows that time is money. There is no need to spend too much of your time or too little of your time preparing for the test. You should only spend as much of your precious time preparing as is necessary for you to get the score you need.

Once you have taken a practice test under real conditions of time constraints, then you will know if you are ready for the test or not.

If you have scored extremely high the first time that you take the practice test, then there is not much point in spending countless hours studying. You are already there.

Benchmark your abilities by retaking practice tests and seeing how much you have improved. Once you consistently score high enough to guarantee success, then you are ready.

If you have scored well below where you need, then knuckle down and begin studying in earnest. Check your improvement regularly through the use of practice tests under real conditions. Above all, don't worry, panic, or give up. The key is perseverance!

Then, when you go to take the test, remain confident and remember how well you did on the practice tests. If you can score high enough on a practice test, then you can do the same on the real thing.

General Strategies

The most important thing you can do is to ignore your fears and jump into the test immediately. Do not be overwhelmed by any strange-sounding terms. You have to jump into the test like jumping into a pool—all at once is the easiest way.

Make Predictions

As you read and understand the question, try to guess what the answer will be. Remember that several of the answer choices are wrong, and once you begin reading them, your mind will immediately become cluttered with answer choices designed to throw you off. Your mind is typically the most focused immediately after you have read the question and digested its contents. If you can, try to predict what the correct answer will be. You may be surprised at what you can predict.

Quickly scan the choices and see if your prediction is in the listed answer choices. If it is, then you can be quite confident that you have the right answer. It still won't hurt to check the other answer choices, but most of the time, you've got it!

Answer the Question

It may seem obvious to only pick answer choices that answer the question, but the test writers can create some excellent answer choices that are wrong. Don't pick an answer just because it sounds right, or you believe it to be true. It MUST answer the question. Once you've made your selection, always go back and check it against the question and make sure that you didn't misread the question and that the answer choice does answer the question posed.

Benchmark

After you read the first answer choice, decide if you think it sounds correct or not. If it doesn't, move on to the next answer choice. If it does, mentally mark that answer choice. This doesn't mean that you've definitely selected it as your answer choice, it just means that it's the best you've seen thus far. Go ahead and read the next choice. If the next choice is worse than the one you've already selected, keep going to the next answer choice. If the next choice is better than the choice you've already selected, mentally mark the new answer choice as your best guess.

The first answer choice that you select becomes your standard. Every other answer choice must be benchmarked against that standard. That choice is correct until proven otherwise by another answer choice beating it out. Once you've decided that no other answer choice seems as good, do one final check to ensure that your answer choice answers the question posed.

Valid Information

Don't discount any of the information provided in the question. Every piece of information may be necessary to determine the correct answer. None of the information in the question is there to throw you off (while the answer choices will certainly have information to throw you off). If two seemingly unrelated topics are discussed, don't ignore either. You can be confident there is a relationship, or it wouldn't be included in the question, and you are probably going to have to determine what is that relationship to find the answer.

Avoid "Fact Traps"

Don't get distracted by a choice that is factually true. Your search is for the answer that answers the question. Stay focused and don't fall for an answer that is true but irrelevant. Always go back to the question and make sure you're choosing an answer that actually answers the question and is not just a true statement. An answer can be factually correct, but it MUST answer the question asked. Additionally, two answers can both be seemingly correct, so be sure to read all of the answer choices, and make sure that you get the one that BEST answers the question.

Milk the Question

Some of the questions may throw you completely off. They might deal with a subject you have not been exposed to, or one that you haven't reviewed in years. While your lack of knowledge about the subject will be a hindrance, the question itself can give you many clues that will help you find the correct answer. Read the question carefully and look for clues. Watch particularly for adjectives and nouns describing difficult terms or words that you don't recognize. Regardless of whether you completely understand a word or not, replacing it with a synonym, either provided or one you more familiar with, may help you to understand what the questions are asking. Rather than wracking your mind about specific detailed information concerning a difficult term or word, try to use mental substitutes that are easier to understand.

The Trap of Familiarity

Don't just choose a word because you recognize it. On difficult questions, you may not recognize a number of words in the answer choices. The test writers don't put "make-believe" words on the test, so don't think that just because you only recognize all the words in one answer choice that that answer choice must be correct. If you only recognize words in one answer choice, then focus on that one. Is it correct? Try your best to determine if it is correct. If it is, that's great. If not, eliminate it. Each word and answer choice you eliminate increases your chances of getting the question correct, even if you then have to guess among the unfamiliar choices.

Eliminate Answers

Eliminate choices as soon as you realize they are wrong. But be careful! Make sure you consider all of the possible answer choices. Just because one appears right, doesn't mean that the next one won't be even better! The test writers will usually put more than one good answer choice for every question, so read all of them. Don't worry if you are stuck between two that seem right. By getting down to just two remaining possible choices, your odds are now 50/50. Rather than wasting too much time, play the odds. You are guessing, but guessing wisely because you've been able to knock out some of the answer choices that you know are wrong. If you are eliminating choices and realize that the last answer choice you are left with is also obviously wrong, don't panic. Start over and consider each choice again. There may easily be something that you missed the first time and will realize on the second pass.

Tough Questions

If you are stumped on a problem or it appears too hard or too difficult, don't waste time. Move on! Remember though, if you can quickly check for obviously incorrect answer choices, your chances of guessing correctly are greatly improved. Before you completely give up, at least try to knock out a couple of possible answers. Eliminate what you can and then guess at the remaining answer choices before moving on.

Brainstorm

If you get stuck on a difficult question, spend a few seconds quickly brainstorming. Run through the complete list of possible answer choices. Look at each choice and ask yourself, "Could this answer the question satisfactorily?" Go through each answer choice and consider it independently of the others. By systematically going through all possibilities, you may find something that you would otherwise overlook. Remember though that when you get stuck, it's important to try to keep moving.

Read Carefully

Understand the problem. Read the question and answer choices carefully. Don't miss the question because you misread the terms. You have plenty of time to read each question thoroughly and make sure you understand what is being asked. Yet a happy medium must be attained, so don't waste too much time. You must read carefully, but efficiently.

Face Value

When in doubt, use common sense. Always accept the situation in the problem at face value. Don't read too much into it. These problems will not require you to make huge leaps of logic. The test writers aren't trying to throw you off with a cheap trick. If you have to go beyond creativity and make a leap of logic in order to have an answer choice answer the question, then you should look at the other answer choices. Don't overcomplicate the problem by creating theoretical relationships or explanations that will warp time or space. These are normal problems rooted in reality. It's just that the applicable relationship or explanation may not be readily apparent and you have to figure things out. Use your common sense to interpret anything that isn't clear.

Prefixes

If you're having trouble with a word in the question or answer choices, try dissecting it. Take advantage of every clue that the word might include. Prefixes and suffixes can be a huge help. Usually they allow you to determine a basic meaning. Pre- means before, post- means after, pro - is positive, de- is negative. From these prefixes and suffixes, you can get an idea of the general meaning of the word and try to put it into context. Beware though of any traps. Just because con- is the opposite of pro-, doesn't necessarily mean congress is the opposite of progress!

Hedge Phrases

Watch out for critical hedge phrases, led off with words such as "likely," "may," "can," "sometimes," "often," "almost," "mostly," "usually," "generally," "rarely," and "sometimes." Question writers insert these hedge phrases to cover every possibility. Often an answer choice will be wrong simply because it leaves no room for exception. Unless the situation calls for them, avoid answer choices that have definitive words like "exactly," and "always."

Switchback Words

Stay alert for "switchbacks." These are the words and phrases frequently used to alert you to shifts in thought. The most common switchback word is "but." Others include "although," "however," "nevertheless," "on the other hand," "even though," "while," "in spite of," "despite," and "regardless of."

New Information

Correct answer choices will rarely have completely new information included. Answer choices typically are straightforward reflections of the material asked about and will directly relate to the question. If a new piece of information is included in an answer choice that doesn't even seem to relate to the topic being asked about, then that answer choice is likely incorrect. All of the information needed to answer the question is usually provided for you in the question. You should not have to make guesses that are unsupported or choose answer choices that require unknown information that cannot be reasoned from what is given.

Time Management

On technical questions, don't get lost on the technical terms. Don't spend too much time on any one question. If you don't know what a term means, then odds are you aren't going to get much further since you don't have a dictionary. You should be able to immediately recognize whether or not you know a term. If you don't, work with the other clues that you have—the other answer choices and terms provided—but don't waste too much time trying to figure out a difficult term that you don't know.

Contextual Clues

Look for contextual clues. An answer can be right but not the correct answer. The contextual clues will help you find the answer that is most right and is correct. Understand the context in which a phrase or statement is made. This will help you make important distinctions.

Don't Panic

Panicking will not answer any questions for you; therefore, it isn't helpful. When you first see the question, if your mind goes blank, take a deep breath. Force yourself to mechanically go through the steps of solving the problem using the strategies you've learned.

Pace Yourself

Don't get clock fever. It's easy to be overwhelmed when you're looking at a page full of questions, your mind is full of random thoughts and feeling confused, and the clock is ticking down faster than you would like. Calm down and maintain the pace that you have set for yourself. As long as you are on track by monitoring your pace, you are guaranteed to have enough time for yourself. When you get to the last few minutes of the test, it may seem like you won't have enough time left, but if you only have as many questions as you should have left at that point, then you're right on track!

Answer Selection

The best way to pick an answer choice is to eliminate all of those that are wrong, until only one is left and confirm that is the correct answer. Sometimes though, an answer choice may immediately look right. Be careful! Take a second to make sure that the other choices are not equally obvious. Don't make a hasty mistake. There are only two times that you should stop before checking other answers. First is when you are positive that the answer choice you have selected is correct. Second is when time is almost out and you have to make a quick guess!

Check Your Work

Since you will probably not know every term listed and the answer to every question, it is important that you get credit for the ones that you do know. Don't miss any questions through careless mistakes. If at all possible, try to take a second to look back over your answer selection and make sure you've selected the correct answer choice and haven't made a costly careless mistake (such as marking an answer choice that you didn't mean to mark). The time it takes for this quick double check should more than pay for itself in caught mistakes.

Beware of Directly Quoted Answers

Sometimes an answer choice will repeat word for word a portion of the question or reference section. However, beware of such exact duplication. It may be a trap! More than likely, the correct choice will paraphrase or summarize a point, rather than being exactly the same wording.

Slang

Scientific sounding answers are better than slang ones. An answer choice that begins "To compare the outcomes..." is much more likely to be correct than one that begins "Because some people insisted..."

Extreme Statements

Avoid wild answers that throw out highly controversial ideas that are proclaimed as established fact. An answer choice that states the "process should used in certain situations, if..." is much more likely to be correct than one that states the "process should be discontinued completely." The first is a calm rational statement and doesn't even make a definitive, uncompromising stance, using a hedge word "if" to provide wiggle room, whereas the second choice is a radical idea and far more extreme.

Answer Choice Families

When you have two or more answer choices that are direct opposites or parallels, one of them is usually the correct answer. For instance, if one answer choice states "x increases" and another answer choice states "x decreases" or "y increases," then those two or three answer choices are very similar in construction and fall into the same family of answer choices. A family of answer choices consists of two or three answer choices, very similar in construction, but often with directly opposite meanings. Usually the correct answer choice will be in that family of answer choices. The "odd man out" or answer choice that doesn't seem to fit the parallel construction of the other answer choices is more likely to be incorrect.

Special Report: What is Test Anxiety and How to Overcome It?

The very nature of tests caters to some level of anxiety, nervousness, or tension, just as we feel for any important event that occurs in our lives. A little bit of anxiety or nervousness can be a good thing. It helps us with motivation, and makes achievement just that much sweeter. However, too much anxiety can be a problem, especially if it hinders our ability to function and perform.

"Test anxiety," is the term that refers to the emotional reactions that some test-takers experience when faced with a test or exam. Having a fear of testing and exams is based upon a rational fear, since the test-taker's performance can shape the course of an academic career. Nevertheless, experiencing excessive fear of examinations will only interfere with the test-taker's ability to perform and chance to be successful.

There are a large variety of causes that can contribute to the development and sensation of test anxiety. These include, but are not limited to, lack of preparation and worrying about issues surrounding the test.

Lack of Preparation

Lack of preparation can be identified by the following behaviors or situations:

Not scheduling enough time to study, and therefore cramming the night before the test or exam
Managing time poorly, to create the sensation that there is not enough time to do everything
Failing to organize the text information in advance, so that the study material consists of the entire text and not simply the pertinent information
Poor overall studying habits

Worrying, on the other hand, can be related to both the test taker, or many other factors around him/her that will be affected by the results of the test. These include worrying about:

Previous performances on similar exams, or exams in general
How friends and other students are achieving
The negative consequences that will result from a poor grade or failure

There are three primary elements to test anxiety. Physical components, which involve the same typical bodily reactions as those to acute anxiety (to be discussed below). Emotional factors have to do with fear or panic. Mental or cognitive issues concerning attention spans and memory abilities.

Physical Signals

There are many different symptoms of test anxiety, and these are not limited to mental and emotional strain. Frequently there are a range of physical signals that will let a test taker know that he/she is suffering from test anxiety. These bodily changes can include the following:

Perspiring
Sweaty palms
Wet, trembling hands
Nausea
Dry mouth
A knot in the stomach
Headache
Faintness
Muscle tension
Aching shoulders, back and neck
Rapid heart beat
Feeling too hot/cold

To recognize the sensation of test anxiety, a test-taker should monitor him/herself for the following sensations:

The physical distress symptoms as listed above
Emotional sensitivity, expressing emotional feelings such as the need to cry or laugh too much, or a sensation of anger or helplessness
A decreased ability to think, causing the test-taker to blank out or have racing thoughts that are hard to organize or control.

Though most students will feel some level of anxiety when faced with a test or exam, the majority can cope with that anxiety and maintain it at a manageable level. However, those who cannot are faced with a very real and very serious condition, which can and should be controlled for the immeasurable benefit of this sufferer.

Naturally, these sensations lead to negative results for the testing experience. The most common effects of test anxiety have to do with nervousness and mental blocking.

Nervousness

Nervousness can appear in several different levels:

The test-taker's difficulty, or even inability to read and understand the questions on the test
The difficulty or inability to organize thoughts to a coherent form
The difficulty or inability to recall key words and concepts relating to the testing questions (especially essays)
The receipt of poor grades on a test, though the test material was well known by the test taker

Conversely, a person may also experience mental blocking, which involves:

Blanking out on test questions
Only remembering the correct answers to the questions when the test has already finished.

Fortunately for test anxiety sufferers, beating these feelings, to a large degree, has to do with proper preparation. When a test taker has a feeling of preparedness, then anxiety will be dramatically lessened.

The first step to resolving anxiety issues is to distinguish which of the two types of anxiety are being suffered. If the anxiety is a direct result of a lack of preparation, this should be considered a normal reaction, and the anxiety level (as opposed to the test results) shouldn't be anything to worry about. However, if, when adequately prepared, the test-taker still panics, blanks out, or seems to overreact, this is not a fully rational reaction. While this can be considered normal too, there are many ways to combat and overcome these effects.

Remember that anxiety cannot be entirely eliminated, however, there are ways to minimize it, to make the anxiety easier to manage. Preparation is one of the best ways to minimize test anxiety. Therefore the following techniques are wise in order to best fight off any anxiety that may want to build.

To begin with, try to avoid cramming before a test, whenever it is possible. By trying to memorize an entire term's worth of information in one day, you'll be shocking your system, and not giving yourself a very good chance to absorb the information. This is an easy path to anxiety, so for those who suffer from test anxiety, cramming should not even be considered an option.

Instead of cramming, work throughout the semester to combine all of the material which is presented throughout the semester, and work on it gradually as the course goes by, making sure to master the main concepts first, leaving minor details for a week or so before the test.

To study for the upcoming exam, be sure to pose questions that may be on the examination, to gauge the ability to answer them by integrating the ideas from your texts, notes and lectures, as well as any supplementary readings.

If it is truly impossible to cover all of the information that was covered in that particular term, concentrate on the most important portions, that can be covered very well. Learn these concepts as best as possible, so that when the test comes, a goal can be made to use these concepts as presentations of your knowledge.

In addition to study habits, changes in attitude are critical to beating a struggle with test anxiety. In fact, an improvement of the perspective over the entire test-taking experience can actually help a test taker to enjoy studying and therefore improve the overall experience. Be certain not to overemphasize the significance of the grade - know that the result of the test is neither a reflection of self worth, nor is it a measure of intelligence; one grade will not predict a person's future success.

To improve an overall testing outlook, the following steps should be tried:

Keeping in mind that the most reasonable expectation for taking a test is to expect to try to demonstrate as much of what you know as you possibly can.
Reminding ourselves that a test is only one test; this is not the only one, and there will be others.
The thought of thinking of oneself in an irrational, all-or-nothing term should be avoided at all costs.
A reward should be designated for after the test, so there's something to look forward to. Whether it be going to a movie, going out to eat, or simply visiting friends, schedule it in advance, and do it no matter what result is expected on the exam.

Test-takers should also keep in mind that the basics are some of the most important things, even beyond anti-anxiety techniques and studying. Never neglect the basic social, emotional and biological needs, in order to try to absorb information. In order to best achieve, these three factors must be held as just as important as the studying itself.

Study Steps

Remember the following important steps for studying:

Maintain healthy nutrition and exercise habits. Continue both your recreational activities and social pass times. These both contribute to your physical and emotional well being.
Be certain to get a good amount of sleep, especially the night before the test, because when you're overtired you are not able to perform to the best of your best ability.
Keep the studying pace to a moderate level by taking breaks when they are needed, and varying the work whenever possible, to keep the mind fresh instead of getting bored.
When enough studying has been done that all the material that can be learned has been learned, and the test taker is prepared for the test, stop studying and do something relaxing such as listening to music, watching a movie, or taking a warm bubble bath.

There are also many other techniques to minimize the uneasiness or apprehension that is experienced along with test anxiety before, during, or even after the examination. In fact, there are a great deal of things that can be done to stop anxiety from interfering with lifestyle and performance. Again, remember that anxiety will not be eliminated entirely, and it shouldn't be. Otherwise that "up" feeling for exams would not exist, and most of us depend on that sensation to perform better than usual. However, this anxiety has to be at a level that is manageable.

Of course, as we have just discussed, being prepared for the exam is half the battle right away. Attending all classes, finding out what knowledge will be expected on the exam, and knowing the exam schedules are easy steps to lowering anxiety. Keeping up with work will remove the need to cram, and efficient study habits will eliminate wasted time. Studying should be done in an ideal location for concentration, so that it is simple to become interested in the material and give it complete attention. A method such as SQ3R (Survey, Question, Read, Recite, Review) is a wonderful key to follow to make sure that the study habits are as effective as possible, especially in the case of learning from a textbook. Flashcards are great techniques for memorization. Learning to take good notes will mean that notes will be full of useful information, so that less sifting will need to be done to seek out what is pertinent for studying. Reviewing notes after class and then again on occasion will keep the information fresh in the mind. From notes that have been taken summary sheets and outlines can be made for simpler reviewing.

A study group can also be a very motivational and helpful place to study, as there will be a sharing of ideas, all of the minds can work together, to make sure that everyone understands, and the studying will be made more interesting because it will be a social occasion.

Basically, though, as long as the test-taker remains organized and self confident, with efficient study habits, less time will need to be spent studying, and higher grades will be achieved.

To become self confident, there are many useful steps. The first of these is "self talk." It has been shown through extensive research, that self-talk for students who suffer from test anxiety, should be well monitored, in order to make sure that it contributes to self confidence as opposed to sinking the student. Frequently the self talk of test-anxious students is negative or self-defeating, thinking that everyone else is smarter and faster, that they always mess up, and that if they don't do well, they'll fail the entire course. It is important to decreasing anxiety that awareness is made of self talk. Try writing any negative self thoughts and then disputing them with a positive statement instead. Begin self-encouragement as though it was a friend speaking. Repeat positive statements to help reprogram the mind to believing in successes instead of failures.

Helpful Techniques

Other extremely helpful techniques include:

Self-visualization of doing well and reaching goals
While aiming for an "A" level of understanding, don't try to "overprotect" by setting your expectations lower. This will only convince the mind to stop studying in order to meet the lower expectations.
Don't make comparisons with the results or habits of other students. These are individual factors, and different things work for different people, causing different results.
Strive to become an expert in learning what works well, and what can be done in order to improve. Consider collecting this data in a journal.
Create rewards for after studying instead of doing things before studying that will only turn into avoidance behaviors.
Make a practice of relaxing - by using methods such as progressive relaxation, self-hypnosis, guided imagery, etc - in order to make relaxation an automatic sensation.
Work on creating a state of relaxed concentration so that concentrating will take on the focus of the mind, so that none will be wasted on worrying.
Take good care of the physical self by eating well and getting enough sleep.
Plan in time for exercise and stick to this plan.

Beyond these techniques, there are other methods to be used before, during and after the test that will help the test-taker perform well in addition to overcoming anxiety.

Before the exam comes the academic preparation. This involves establishing a study schedule and beginning at least one week before the actual date of the test. By doing this, the anxiety of not having enough time to study for the test will be automatically eliminated. Moreover, this will make the studying a much more effective experience, ensuring that the learning will be an easier process. This relieves much undue pressure on the test-taker.

Summary sheets, note cards, and flash cards with the main concepts and examples of these main concepts should be prepared in advance of the actual studying time. A topic should never be eliminated from this process. By omitting a topic because it isn't expected to be on the test is only setting up the test-taker for anxiety should it actually appear on the exam. Utilize the course syllabus for laying out the topics that should be studied. Carefully go over the notes that were made in class, paying special attention to any of the issues that the professor took special care to emphasize while lecturing in class. In the textbooks, use the chapter review, or if possible, the chapter tests, to begin your review.

It may even be possible to ask the instructor what information will be covered on the exam, or what the format of the exam will be (for example, multiple choice, essay, free form, true-false). Additionally, see if it is possible to find out how many questions will be on the test. If a review sheet or sample test has been offered by the professor, make good use of it, above anything else, for the preparation for the test. Another great resource for getting to know the examination is reviewing tests from previous semesters. Use these tests to review, and aim to achieve a 100% score on each of the possible topics. With a few exceptions, the goal that you set for yourself is the highest one that you will reach.

Take all of the questions that were assigned as homework, and rework them to any other possible course material. The more problems reworked, the more skill and confidence will form as a result. When forming the solution to a problem, write out each of the steps. Don't simply do head work. By doing as many steps on paper as possible, much clarification and therefore confidence will be formed. Do this with as many homework problems as possible, before checking the answers. By checking the answer after each problem, a reinforcement will exist, that will not be on the exam. Study situations should be as exam-like as possible, to prime the test-taker's system for the experience. By waiting to check the answers at the end, a psychological advantage will be formed, to decrease the stress factor.

Another fantastic reason for not cramming is the avoidance of confusion in concepts, especially when it comes to mathematics. 8-10 hours of study will become one hundred percent more effective if it is spread out over a week or at least several days, instead of doing it all in one sitting. Recognize that the human brain requires time in order to assimilate new material, so frequent breaks and a span of study time over several days will be much more beneficial.

Additionally, don't study right up until the point of the exam. Studying should stop a minimum of one hour before the exam begins. This allows the brain to rest and put things in their proper order. This will also provide the time to become as relaxed as possible when going into the examination room. The test-taker will also have time to eat well and eat sensibly. Know that the brain needs food as much as the rest of the body. With enough food and enough sleep, as well as a relaxed attitude, the body and the mind are primed for success.

Avoid any anxious classmates who are talking about the exam. These students only spread anxiety, and are not worth sharing the anxious sentimentalities.

Before the test also involves creating a positive attitude, so mental preparation should also be a point of concentration. There are many keys to creating a positive attitude. Should fears become rushing in, make a visualization of taking the exam, doing well, and seeing an A written on the paper. Write out a list of affirmations that will bring a feeling of confidence, such as "I am doing well in my English class," "I studied well and know my material," "I enjoy this class." Even if the affirmations aren't believed at first, it sends a positive message to the subconscious which will result in an alteration of the overall belief system, which is the system that creates reality.

If a sensation of panic begins, work with the fear and imagine the very worst! Work through the entire scenario of not passing the test, failing the entire course, and dropping out of school, followed by not getting a job, and pushing a shopping cart through the dark alley where you'll live. This will place things into perspective! Then, practice deep breathing and create a visualization of the opposite situation - achieving an "A" on the exam, passing the entire course, receiving the degree at a graduation ceremony.

On the day of the test, there are many things to be done to ensure the best results, as well as the most calm outlook. The following stages are suggested in order to maximize test-taking potential:

Begin the examination day with a moderate breakfast, and avoid any coffee or beverages with caffeine if the test taker is prone to jitters. Even people who are used to managing caffeine can feel jittery or light-headed when it is taken on a test day.
Attempt to do something that is relaxing before the examination begins. As last minute cramming clouds the mastering of overall concepts, it is better to use this time to create a calming outlook.
Be certain to arrive at the test location well in advance, in order to provide time to select a location that is away from doors, windows and other distractions, as well as giving enough time to relax before the test begins.
Keep away from anxiety generating classmates who will upset the sensation of stability and relaxation that is being attempted before the exam.
Should the waiting period before the exam begins cause anxiety, create a self-distraction by reading a light magazine or something else that is relaxing and simple.

During the exam itself, read the entire exam from beginning to end, and find out how much time should be allotted to each individual problem. Once writing the exam, should more time be taken for a problem, it should be abandoned, in order to begin

- 150 -

another problem. If there is time at the end, the unfinished problem can always be returned to and completed.

Read the instructions very carefully - twice - so that unpleasant surprises won't follow during or after the exam has ended.

When writing the exam, pretend that the situation is actually simply the completion of homework within a library, or at home. This will assist in forming a relaxed atmosphere, and will allow the brain extra focus for the complex thinking function.

Begin the exam with all of the questions with which the most confidence is felt. This will build the confidence level regarding the entire exam and will begin a quality momentum. This will also create encouragement for trying the problems where uncertainty resides.

Going with the "gut instinct" is always the way to go when solving a problem. Second guessing should be avoided at all costs. Have confidence in the ability to do well.

For essay questions, create an outline in advance that will keep the mind organized and make certain that all of the points are remembered. For multiple choice, read every answer, even if the correct one has been spotted - a better one may exist.

Continue at a pace that is reasonable and not rushed, in order to be able to work carefully. Provide enough time to go over the answers at the end, to check for small errors that can be corrected.

Should a feeling of panic begin, breathe deeply, and think of the feeling of the body releasing sand through its pores. Visualize a calm, peaceful place, and include all of the sights, sounds and sensations of this image. Continue the deep breathing, and take a few minutes to continue this with closed eyes. When all is well again, return to the test.

If a "blanking" occurs for a certain question, skip it and move on to the next question. There will be time to return to the other question later. Get everything done that can be done, first, to guarantee all the grades that can be compiled, and to build all of the confidence possible. Then return to the weaker questions to build the marks from there.

Remember, one's own reality can be created, so as long as the belief is there, success will follow. And remember: anxiety can happen later, right now, there's an exam to be written!

After the examination is complete, whether there is a feeling for a good grade or a bad grade, don't dwell on the exam, and be certain to follow through on the reward that was promised…and enjoy it! Don't dwell on any mistakes that have been made, as there is nothing that can be done at this point anyway.

Additionally, don't begin to study for the next test right away. Do something relaxing for a while, and let the mind relax and prepare itself to begin absorbing information again.

From the results of the exam - both the grade and the entire experience, be certain to learn from what has gone on. Perfect studying habits and work some more on confidence in order to make the next examination experience even better than the last one.

Learn to avoid places where openings occurred for laziness, procrastination and day dreaming.

Use the time between this exam and the next one to better learn to relax, even learning to relax on cue, so that any anxiety can be controlled during the next exam. Learn how to relax the body. Slouch in your chair if that helps. Tighten and then relax all of the different muscle groups, one group at a time, beginning with the feet and then working all the way up to the neck and face. This will ultimately relax the muscles more than they were to begin with. Learn how to breathe deeply and comfortably, and focus on this breathing going in and out as a relaxing thought. With every exhale, repeat the word "relax."

As common as test anxiety is, it is very possible to overcome it. Make yourself one of the test-takers who overcome this frustrating hindrance.

Special Report: Additional Bonus Material

Due to our efforts to try to keep this book to a manageable length, we've created a link that will give you access to all of your additional bonus material.

Please visit http://www.mometrix.com/bonus948/patientcare to access the information.